S. Hrg. 110–26

THE PHYSICIAN SHORTAGE CRISIS IN RURAL AMERICA: WHO WILL TREAT OUR PATIENTS?

FIELD HEARING

OF THE

COMMITTEE ON HEALTH, EDUCATION, LABOR, AND PENSIONS

UNITED STATES SENATE

ONE HUNDRED TENTH CONGRESS

FIRST SESSION

ON

EXAMINING THE PHYSICIAN SHORTAGE CRISIS IN RURAL AMERICA, FOCUSING ON ACCESS TO HEALTH CARE IN ALASKA

FEBRUARY 20, 2007 (ANCHORAGE, AK)

Printed for the use of the Committee on Health, Education, Labor, and Pensions

Available via the World Wide Web: http://www.gpoaccess.gov/congress/senate

U.S. GOVERNMENT PRINTING OFFICE

33–768 PDF   WASHINGTON : 2007

For sale by the Superintendent of Documents, U.S. Government Printing Office
Internet: bookstore.gpo.gov   Phone: toll free (866) 512–1800; DC area (202) 512–1800
Fax: (202) 512–2104   Mail: Stop IDCC, Washington, DC 20402–0001

(II)

CONTENTS

STATEMENTS

TUESDAY, FEBRUARY 20, 2007

(III)

FIELD HEARING
THE PHYSICIAN SHORTAGE CRISIS IN RURAL AMERICA: WHO WILL TREAT OUR PATIENTS

TUESDAY, FEBRUARY 20, 2007

U.S. SENATE,
COMMITTEE ON HEALTH, EDUCATION, LABOR, AND PENSIONS,
Anchorage, AK.

The committee met, pursuant to notice, at 9 a.m., at the Loussac Public Library, 3600 Denali Street, Anchorage, Alaska, Hon. Lisa Murkowski, presiding.

Present: Senator Murkowski.

OPENING STATEMENT OF SENATOR MURKOWSKI

Senator MURKOWSKI. We'll call to order the field hearing for the Health, Education, Labor, and Pensions Committee.

I'd like to welcome you all here this morning to talk about an issue that is of great concern to us here in this State, and truly to Americans across the country, particularly in those more rural areas.

Just a little bit of process here before we begin this morning. We do have a set witness list of invited participants that we have asked to address this issue. I do believe that you should have received a copy of that when you signed in. I do understand this morning that there are some individuals who would like the opportunity to give their perspective on physician access here in the State of Alaska. While we had not anticipated that, I would welcome the opportunity to hear your comments. So, the revised plan—if you will—this morning, is that we'll have the opportunity for individuals to make a short statement at the conclusion of the panelists' testimony.

If you chose not to provide your statement orally here today, we would encourage you to submit your statements in writing. They will be made part of the Health, Education, Labor, and Pensions Committee record. So, that will be part of the committee's deliberation as we take the issue up back in Washington, DC.

So, whether you choose to submit your comment here this morning, or in writing—your choice—we'll hold the record open on this for a 2-week period, so if you would like to submit those comments, you may do so in writing.

Maggie Elehwany, who is just walking off here, is my legislative assistant on healthcare matters, and she would be the contact person for those of you who might have any questions as to the process.

As I've indicated, this is a HELP Committee Field Hearing, I do believe it's probably the first such hearing that we've ever had in this State. I am the first of Alaska's Senators to serve on this committee, a committee of very important jurisdiction to all of us. So, to have the opportunity this morning, as Alaskans, to put our comments on the record for my colleagues back in Washington to see and understand our situation, I think is very important. And I am most appreciative to the Chairman of the committee, Senator Kennedy, and the Ranking Member, Senator Enzi, for allowing us to have this, this morning.

Now, some have asked me, "Well, why are we even having this field hearing up here? What's going on up in Alaska?" And, I will start off by reading just a few snips from some e-mails that I have received from constituents, and this is just kind of random sampling out of the correspondence files as they come in.

Over the past year, the volume of e-mails, faxes, letters saying, "I can't find a doctor to care for me. I cannot find—I cannot get an appointment as a Medicare-eligible patient, what do I do?"

I've got one here from a constituent here in Anchorage, who says,

> "My mother has returned to Alaska to retire near her grandchildren, and has had difficulty in the extreme in getting a doctor who will take her, as she is a Medicare patient. My mother has made in excess of 100 calls to physicians in Anchorage."

Another woman from Anchorage writes,

> "During the past year, I've tried to find a doctor that accepts Medicare. I used the Anchorage Yellow Pages and called over 100 doctors, only to be told that they won't accept any more Medicare patients. I'll tell you ahead of time, we'll be going to the hospital emergency rooms to receive even the basic medical care for colds and flu and other basic needs that could have been treated by seeing a doctor at their established practice. This doesn't sound like good fiscal management."

Another letter, one that was actually reprinted in the *Anchorage Daily News* from a person here in Anchorage, says "My friend's telephoned more than 80 doctors recently, and no one was accepting new Medicare patients." Another constituent from Kenai writes,

> "My mom has Medicare, and she had to wait 5 months to be seen by a neurologist, because she'd been put on a waiting list to be seen, due to the fact that she was a Medicare patient."

E-mail after e-mail, fax after fax, phone call after phone call, saying, "What do we do? Whom do I go to? How long is the list? What can we do?" And so, it's comments like these from constituents all over the State that has precipitated the need for this hearing today.

And I will tell you, we will focus here today on the Alaska situation, but we must also keep in mind that, as we face the challenges here, in Alaska, Americans across the country in rural parts of the Nation are facing similar concerns.

Patients cannot access healthcare because of the dangerously low shortages of healthcare providers. In just 20 years, 20 percent of the U.S. population will be 65 years, or older, and this will be a larger percentage than in any time in our Nation's history. And just as this aging population places the highest demands on our healthcare system, we've got some experts that are predicting a national shortage of 200,000 physicians. If that becomes a reality, 84 million patients will be without a doctor's care.

There's already a dozen States—including Alaska, now—that report physician shortages. And the shortages exist in radiology, cardiology, neurology, just to name a few, but the greatest shortages persistently have been in primary care. In fact, the shortage of primary care physicians in rural areas of the United States represents one of the most intractable health policy problems of the past century.

So, the question is, Where are the doctors going? What's happening out there? And we're losing our doctors through attrition—one-third of physicians are 55 years or older, and are likely to retire just as this baby boom generation moves into its time of greatest medical need. Additionally, for the last quarter of a century, medical schools have kept their student enrollments virtually flat, so we're not seeing the medical students coming out.

But, we're also losing our doctors to frustration. Low Medicaid and Medicare reimbursement rates, coupled with complex regulations and paperwork, leave physicians aggravated and disappointed with the practice of medicine.

We'll hear from one of our witnesses this morning that Medicaid—which covers nearly one in five Alaskans, and one in three Alaskan children, once again, will receive cuts in Federal dollars if the temporary formula is not extended or made permanent.

The recent Federal reductions in Alaska Medicare reimbursement rates have been so severe, that our physicians report reimbursement rates are only about 40 percent of the actual cost of treating patients. Losing money by seeing Medicare patients has meant that many, many physicians have stopped accepting Medicare patients entirely. And, this was reflected in the frustration of some of the e-mails that I read to you.

We hear the stories from seniors all over the State who call physician after physician, but they can't find a doctor who's willing to accept them. And, if you are lucky enough to find a physician, it often may take weeks or months to get an appointment. And, when faced with that kind of a delay, patients essentially have one of two options—they go to the emergency room, or they don't go at all.

In rural America, patients have long gone without care. Despite the fact that one-fifth of the U.S. population lives in rural America, only 9 percent of our Nation's physicians are practicing in these areas. Over 50 million of these rural Americans live in areas that have a shortage of physicians to meet basic needs.

Physician recruitment in rural America is a problem. High student debt often forces many students away from rural practice, and into urban-specialty medicine. In Alaska, we know that the definition of rural here is a little bit different than in the Lower 48. But, our definition of rural, and how we deal with that, and you compound that with the physician shortage crisis, and the situation is just magnified.

Right now, Alaska has the sixth lowest ratio of physicians to population in the United States. Once you go outside the Anchorage area, we're dead last. In other words, outside of Anchorage, the physician to population ratio is the worst in the Nation.

Now, while we don't have a medical school here in this State, we do have two successful programs that have helped train Alaskans as physicians, or to help bring doctors to the State. This is the University of Washington Medical School program, known as WWAMI, we also have the Alaska Family Physician Residency Program.

But, despite the success of these two great programs, we recognize the inadequacies in that each of them are far too small to meet the population's needs. In fact, the State has clearly recognized the crisis that we are facing, and last year the University of Alaska, in conjunction with the State, established a task force. We'll hear some of the details from that task force presented to us today, and we greatly appreciate that.

The challenge that we face, that our seniors face, and others face, who don't have access to a doctor—it's an unacceptable situation. We must help current physicians stay in the practice of medicine, and we must vastly increase our healthcare workforce.

Senator Stevens and I have been working together to fight for fair Medicaid and Medicare reimbursement rates for Alaskan providers. I've introduced the Rural Physician Relief Act; this is a bill that provides tax incentives for physicians to practice in our most rural and our frontier locations. I'm also going to be introducing a bill when we get back to Washington after this President's Day recess, this will be the Physician Shortage Elimination Act, and what this will essentially provide for is to double the funding for the National Health Service Corporation.

It will equally allow rural and underserved residency programs to expand, by removing barriers that prevent the programs from developing rural training rotations, and will create programs that target disadvantaged youth in rural and underserved areas. Essentially, it will create a pipeline to careers in healthcare. And finally, to bolster the cornerstone of rural healthcare, which is the community health center, through grants, and by allowing them to expand their residency programs.

There's a great deal that we must do, but today, this is my opportunity to hear from you about the specifics on the ground here in this State, and again, so that I can take that back to Washington to help explain to others why we need to act, and act quickly, as we address access to healthcare here in this State.

And with that introduction, I would like to bring up on the first panel, we have Karleen Jackson, who is the Commissioner of the State Department of Health and Social Services. Commissioner Jackson has been very instrumental, as we have worked on Medicare and Medicaid issues, and I appreciate you coming this morning, Commissioner, up from Juneau to provide the perspective.

And, with that, if you would like to proceed.

STATEMENT OF KARLEEN JACKSON, COMMISSIONER, STATE DEPARTMENT OF HEALTH AND SOCIAL SERVICES, JUNEAU, ALASKA

Ms. JACKSON. Thank you, Senator Murkowski. I'd also like to thank the committee for allowing Alaska to host this important field hearing to talk about healthcare access in rural America.

My written testimony provides references to several important facts that are in the written materials, many of which are out on the table, that outline the issues that compound the rural healthcare crisis in Alaska, as you so eloquently explained in your introduction.

Some of the facts, for example, there are just over 670,000 people living across more than 570 square miles in Alaska. One hundred and fifty-two thousand people in 230 villages and communities—including our capital city—only are able to access services outside their area by air or water transportation, weather and conditions permitting.

The annual cost of recruitment of healthcare workers in Alaska was over $24 million in 2005–2006, with $15 million attributable to rural facilities. Average cost per physician hired were over $74,000, with rural costs per hire 44 percent higher than urban.

Healthcare costs in Alaska are 70 percent higher than those in the Lower 48. In 2004, 16 percent of rural Alaskan physician positions were vacant, and shortages are expected to increase over the next 20 years, as the State's population ages, and physicians retire.

As mentioned, the number of people 65 and older in Alaska is projected to increase from 43,000 to 124,000 people between 2005 and 2025. This will exacerbate the problems created by the expiration on January 1, 2006 of the Medicare Physician Reimbursement Formula, that had helped encourage Alaskan physicians to accept Medicare patients.

Medicaid provides healthcare coverage for nearly one in five Alaskan residents, including almost one in three children, making Medicaid the second-largest healthcare insurance payer in the State. Alaska has the largest Native American population served by Medicaid in the Nation, with 52,000, or nearly 40 percent American Indian or Alaskan Native enrollees in fiscal year 2005.

Alaska's frontier and rural areas have the largest number of people requiring Federal healthcare assistance. As a result, several Federal funding issues will significantly compound the problems, with access to healthcare in Alaska, unless they're addressed by Congress.

The Deficit Reduction Act of 2005, set the Alaska Federal Medicare Assistance Formula, or FMAP percent rate, at 57.58 percent until September 30, 2007, at which time it reverts to the formula-derived rate of 52.48 percent. However, the formula reduction does not take into account Alaska's high cost of care, especially for those Alaskans living in areas of the State that experience Third World conditions, and for which physician recruitment issues are exacerbated.

It is critical to the success of the Alaska-Denali Kid Care Program, not only that Federal SCHIP be reauthorized, but also that the funding formula be changed, so that Alaska is not dependent on the redistributed funds from other States to ensure access to healthcare for the one in three Alaskan children who rely on this program.

And the Federal Continuing Resolution has had a negative impact upon tribal healthcare corporations, by reducing funding for some at a time when already high fuel prices are rising, resulting in some corporations actually securing short-term loans to maintain services.

In conclusion, the shortage of physicians in Alaska, particularly in our rural and frontier areas of Alaska, must be addressed within the context of our larger healthcare system challenges, including shortages of other healthcare professionals and para-professionals, and funding decreases across several Federal sources.

We appreciate Congressional support for efforts such as the Dental Health Aid Therapist Program that helps Alaska meet our healthcare needs, and Senator Murkowski, with you, to solve the physician shortage crisis in our Nation and in our State.

Thank you for allowing us an opportunity to bring this issue to the attention of the HELP Committee.

[The prepared statement of Ms. Jackson follows:]

PREPARED STATEMENT OF KARLEEN JACKSON

Thank you for allowing Alaska to host this important field hearing to discuss access to healthcare in rural America. And, thank you, Senator Lisa Murkowski, for your strong support for finding solutions to meet the healthcare needs of Alaskans, particularly those living in rural and frontier areas of our vast State.

According to data from the Alaska Department of Labor and Workforce Development, there are 670,053 people (Census Bureau and Alaska official estimates for 2006) living across the 570,374 square miles that make up our State. Connected by a road system are 518,000 people—weather and conditions permitting—while 152,000 people in 230 villages and communities (including Juneau, our Capital city) can only access services outside their area by air or water transportation

The Status of Recruitment Resources and Strategies (SORRAS II) report published in June 2006 found the annual cost of recruitment of healthcare workers in Alaska was over $24 million in 2005–2006, with $15 million attributable to rural facilities. Average costs per physician hired were over $74,000, with rural costs per hire 44 percent higher than urban.

These facts help to explain some of the reasons the healthcare costs in Alaska are 70 percent higher than those in the contiguous States of the United States. However, a number of studies and reports have been produced in the last few years to help further quantify the scope of the challenges we face in creating an affordable, accessible healthcare delivery system in Alaska.

In January 2006, University of Alaska President, Mark Hamilton and I commissioned the Alaska Physician Supply Task Force to identify the current and future need for physicians in Alaska, as well as strategies to meet those needs. The Task Force Report, published in August 2006 identified that 16 percent of rural Alaskan physician positions were vacant in 2004, with the shortages of physicians expected to increase over the next 20 years as the State's population ages and physicians retire. The aging of Alaska's population impacts our physician shortage in other ways, as well.

According to the 2006 Long Term Forecast produced by the Lewin Group and ECONorthwest, the number of people 65 and older in Alaska is projected to increase from 43,000 to 124,000 between 2005 and 2025. This will exacerbate the problems created by the expiration on January 1, 2006 of the Medicare physician reimbursement formula that had helped encourage Alaskan physicians to accept Medicare patients. Inadequate Medicare rate reimbursements for physicians must be addressed both to encourage physicians to come to Alaska and to support their ability to care for elderly patients.

The Medicaid Program Review commissioned by the Alaska Senate Finance Committee and published in January 2007 reported that Medicaid provides healthcare coverage for nearly one in five Alaskan residents, including one in three children—making Medicaid the second largest health insurance payer in the State, while it ranks third nationally. Furthermore, Alaska has the largest Native American population served by Medicaid in the Nation, with 52,000 American Indian or Alaska Native enrollees in fiscal year 2005—representing nearly 40 percent of Alaskan Medicaid recipients.

Several Federal funding issues will significantly impact access to healthcare for low-income Alaskans unless they are addressed by Congress. First, the Deficit Reduction Act of 2005 set the Alaska Federal Medicaid Assistance Percentage (FMAP) rate at 57.58 percent until September 30, 2007, at which time it will revert to the formula derived rate of 52.48 percent. However, the formula reduction does not take into account Alaska's high cost of care, instead considering only the relative personal income of Alaska residents compared to the national average. A reduction in Alaska's FMAP rate would decrease the Federal Government's ongoing contribution and commitment to Alaska's Medicaid program—requiring an estimated $37 million in State general funds for the 9 months of State fiscal year 2008, and even greater levels of State general funding in future years.

In addition to the FMAP rate decrease, it should also be noted that President Bush's 2008 budget proposal requests that Medicaid administrative funding be reduced to 50 percent. Some current administrative activities, such as Medicaid Management Information System (MMIS) procurement is funded at 90 percent Federal Medicaid; with other administrative activities at 75 percent. Estimates are that a drop to 50 percent in administrative funding would result in an additional loss of $14 million for Alaska. Widely fluctuating matching proportions severely impact budget stability for the department and hinder our ability to plan and fund future healthcare services.

Federal SCHIP funds support Alaska's Denali KidCare program—an important component of Alaska's healthcare system. However, it is critical to the success of this program, not only that SCHIP be reauthorized, but also that the funding formula be changed so that Alaska is not dependent on the redistributed funds from other States to ensure access to healthcare for low-income children and families. Reauthorization that does not address the inequities of the current funding formula will severely disadvantage Alaska by reducing our ability to fund Denali KidCare.

The Federal Continuing Resolution (CR) that has funded Federal programs in lieu of budget bills has had a negative impact upon tribal healthcare corporations. In a usual year the annual Indian Health Service grant to tribes would increase by 1 to 2 percent and the payment would be received such that Alaska tribes could gain interest on the grant amount. This year the CR provided installment payments to tribes at Federal fiscal year 2006 level, which included a 1 percent rescission. This decreased level of funding has resulted in many of the Alaska tribal health corporations securing short-term loans to maintain services, thus paying interest rather than earning interest. Certainly, not all tribal fiscal challenges are a result of the CR process—however, the current CR situation compounds other challenges such as the very high cost of energy in rural Alaska.

Several efforts are underway to address the challenges Alaska faces in recruiting and retaining physicians—especially in rural areas. For example, workforce development strategies outlined in the Physician Supply Task Force report (2006) which Congress could support include: Federal loan repayment programs which play a major role in bringing doctors and other providers to Alaska; support for the National Health Service Corps and the Indian Health Service; expansion of medical school classes, and funding for residency programs and teaching hospital activities can help improve Alaska's recruitment opportunities as well as support the national supply; and support for Senator Murkowski's proposal for a tax credit for physicians agreeing to practice in frontier areas would improve the situation for Alaska.

The Alaska Senate Finance Committee's recently released Medicaid Program Review (January 2007) provides useful guidance and information about policy and funding options including potential 1115 Waiver options which are currently under development to increase Alaska's strategies for improving prevention and disease management to save future healthcare costs.

Governor Sarah Palin, through Administrative Order No. 232 dated February 15, 2007, created the Alaska Health Care Strategies Council to develop an action plan for Alaska to ensure access to quality, affordable healthcare. This Council will compile and analyze the current components of the healthcare system in Alaska; review the various planning reports compiled to address the gaps in service; develop short-term and long-term statewide strategies to improve healthcare access, control cost, and ensure quality of care; and draft performance measures to assess the success of implementing those strategies. Public involvement and input will be included as the Council prepares an action plan for the Governor and legislature by January 2008.

Finally, we appreciate the congressional support for the Alaska Native Tribal Health Consortium's Dental Health Aide Therapist program, as well as the funding efforts that support the healthcare delivery system in Alaska including: HRSA funding for the Community Health Centers program, National Health Services Corps, Rural Hospital Flexibility Program, Small Hospital Improvement Program, State Office of Rural Health, Outreach and Network Grants; USDHHS funding from the: Centers for Disease Control and Prevention, National Institutes of Health, and SAMHSA. These Federal funds work together to support rural health facilities, pandemic flu preparedness, obesity and diabetes management and prevention, fetal alcohol syndrome treatment and prevention, HIV/AIDS monitoring, oral health, cardiovascular disease management, tobacco-related illness reduction, EMS services,

Residential Psychiatric Treatment Centers, Behavioral Health Aides, suicide prevention efforts, disease and risk surveillance, and State planning efforts to increase healthcare coverage for the uninsured.

In conclusion, the shortage of physicians in Alaska—particularly in our rural and frontier areas must be addressed within the context of our larger healthcare system challenges—including shortages of other healthcare professionals and para-professionals and funding decreases across several Federal sources.*

*Sources: Alaska DHSS, Status of Recruitment Resources and Strategies 2005–2006 (SORRAS II). June 2006; Alaska Physician Supply Task Force, Securing an Adequate Number of Physicians for Alaska's Needs. August 2006; Alaska Department of Labor and Workforce Development, Alaska Population Estimates online at *www.labor.state.ak.us.*; Lewin Group and ECONorthwest, Medicaid Long Term Forecast; and Pacific Health Policy Group, Medicaid Program Review, January 2007.

Senator MURKOWSKI. Thank you, Commissioner. I appreciate your comments and the good work that you do in this area.

You've indicated the impact to the State—the financial impact to the State—as a consequence of the Federal Medicaid Assistance Percentage, the FMAP. And, as we look, the financial hit—you've indicated it's about $37 million in State General Funds this year, but with the potential for an additional $14 million if, in fact, the proposal should go ahead to do further reductions.

We can understand what the numbers look like on the ledger, we know that that's going to be a huge hit to the State. But, what does that do within your Department, should the State have to assume that financial hit, because of the reduction—what's that going to do to your budget, within the Department of Health and Social Services?

Ms. JACKSON. Senator Murkowski, what it would do for our budget in the Department, would have serious consequences for access to care, and quality of care, for Alaskans. We've done, I believe, a pretty remarkable job over the last several years of tightening up, as much as possible, every dollar that we spend, every Medicaid dollar coming in, and at this point in time, those kinds of reductions would mean reductions to services for Alaskans. And when we look at those reductions in light of the physician supply shortage, and other workforce development issues, the combination is somewhat the perfect storm. That would mean that Alaskans are not going to get the healthcare that they need.

Senator MURKOWSKI. So, in other words, if people think the situation is bad now, they can anticipate that it will be worse, should these reductions continue.

Ms. JACKSON. That's correct.

Senator MURKOWSKI. Let me ask about the task force that the State commissioned with the University, to analyze the physician shortage problems. The report is pretty specific in its conclusion that there will be significant consequences for access, and for quality of care. But, do you also see that costs would continue to increase, as a result of the squeeze, if you will, or the constriction to access?

Ms. JACKSON. Absolutely. One of the biggest problems, and you mentioned this in your introduction, is when people don't have appropriate healthcare—don't have access to appropriate healthcare— they wind up being seen in emergency rooms at a much higher cost than they would otherwise be seen. And, so every dollar that we're not able to put into preventive care costs us more money, in the long run, when people have to be seen for those higher care costs.

Senator MURKOWSKI. And, I would imagine that many of our systems are already overwhelmed when it comes to providing that level of service that is necessary in the emergency rooms.

Ms. JACKSON. That would be absolutely true.

Senator MURKOWSKI. As we look at the demographics of this State, and recognize that we have an aging population—we're seeing the numbers of physicians dropping—is Alaska prepared to meet its healthcare needs?

Ms. JACKSON. Senator Murkowski, I don't believe we are. I believe it's critical that we have these kinds of conversations right now, the Governor is also—through Administrative Order—created a Healthcare Strategies Council, which I believe will help us in the next year to look at these issues. But, if we don't address these issues in the next few months, or at least the next year, I'm very concerned about what that's going to mean for health in Alaska. And I know I'm not alone in that, and you'll hear that from many other people.

But it is a time when many things are converging to create a crisis of healthcare for Alaskans.

Senator MURKOWSKI. Well, we would look forward to hearing the outcome from the Council that has been recently formed, and there are many different entities, whether it's the Task Force, or the newly appointed Council. We're going to be speaking this afternoon to the roundtable on healthcare that has been pulled together by Commonwealth North. There are a great many entities that are discussing the problem. But, we've got to get beyond the discussions stage, and say, "How are we going to be answering some of these concerns that we are highlighting?" So, I look forward to working with you on this council, and sharing some of the information that we gain.

Ms. JACKSON. Thank you, Senator Murkowski. I look forward to that, too, and we hope that that will roll up all of the good planning that's been done, and come out with an actual action plan for Alaska.

Senator MURKOWSKI. Thank you. I appreciate you coming here this morning, and providing us with your testimony.

With that, I would like to welcome to the second panel, Mrs. Rita Hatch, who is with the Older Persons Action Group; Mr. Frank Appel, who is Chair of the Alaska Commission on Aging; and I'm also going to invite up Mr. Carl Berger, who is the Executive Director of the Lower Kuskokwim Economic Development Council, out of Bethel, Alaska.

And, you all don't need to crowd on to one table there, if you want to have more room, you may, but if you want to huddle together for warmth, I'm okay with that, too.

[Laughter.]

Again, I welcome you all to the committee, and I thank you for your advocacy on behalf of Alaska's seniors, and with that, Mrs. Hatch, why don't we begin with you?

STATEMENT OF RITA HATCH, OLDER PERSONS ACTION GROUP, INCORPORATED, ANCHORAGE, ALASKA

Ms. HATCH. Good morning, Senator, thank you for inviting me here.

I'm a volunteer with the Older Persons Action Group, and I'm well-versed in Medicare, Medicaid, Social Security and other senior issues. And as such, I advocate for seniors in Alaska.

The most important issue facing seniors in Alaska today, is finding a physician who will take the most new Medicare patients, you know that. But what good is having a prescription drug program, if you can't find a doctor to write a prescription?

And what good is paying for Medicare Part B, which pays for doctor's services, if you can't find a doctor to serve you?

With the assistance of some of the staff at OPAG, I have an ongoing telephone survey of medical facilities in Anchorage, to find out which ones of them will take new Medicare patients. And I receive approximately 10 calls a week from seniors who don't have a doctor, and have tried and tried, and finally get around to calling me, and the only thing I can tell them to do is to see a nurse practitioner. I do have a list of nurse practitioners who take care of new Medicare patients.

There's only one clinic in Anchorage that I know of who is taking new Medicare patients, and that's the Anchorage Neighborhood Health Center. The Providence Family Clinic can't take any more, they haven't taken any more for months now. And, there are about 20 doctors that I know of, outside of the clinics, who are taking new Medicare patients, of all of the doctors in Anchorage.

I have one senior who called me the other day—she's still working, and she's working for a big company who has insurance. But she's 65, and her doctor told her he will not take her. Even though Medicare is secondary, he still won't take her. So, I don't know what his reasoning is, because the insurance would pay most of it, anyway.

Then I have another man who just called me the other day, he's 63, and his doctor said to him the other day, "When you're 65, I'm not taking you any more." And he just called me up and said, "What is going on?"

So, this is the situation, I get people calling who bring parents up from outside who tell me the same story, they can't find a doctor. Of course, my temporary solution is the nurse practitioners, but I think there's got to be something else. It seems to me the State of Alaska should be offering incentives for doctors to come up here, to practice up here, and not just in—well, we need them in the rural areas, but we need them in Anchorage, too.

I have talked to people in other States, and we seem to be the worst of them. Montana has the same problem, I don't know what other States do, but those are the two States who have a big problem, and it's because of the low population, I guess.

But, it's up to you, to get us some help here, please.

[Laughter.]

There aren't many seniors in the audience today, besides me, and I really don't have a dog in this fight, because I'm a retiree from the State, and I have good insurance, and I am a patient at Anchorage Neighborhood Health Center. But I'm here to advocate for the people who don't have any help.

[The prepared statement of Ms. Hatch follows:]

PREPARED STATEMENT OF RITA HATCH

My name is Rita Hatch. I am a volunteer with the Older Persons Action Group. I am well versed in Medicare, Medicaid, Social Security and other Senior issues and as such, I advocate for seniors in Alaska.

The most important issue facing seniors in Alaska today is finding a physician who will take them as new Medicare patients. What good is having a prescription drug program in Medicare if you can't find a doctor to write a prescription? What good is paying for Medicare Part B, if you can't find a doctor to treat you?

With the assistance of some staff at OPAG, I have an ongoing telephone survey of the medical facilities in Anchorage, to ascertain, which of them will take new Medicare patients.

I have one senior, who is still working and has insurance and she still can't find a doctor to treat her, although in her case, Medicare would be the secondary payer of her bill.

I receive approximately 10 calls a week from seniors who are trying to find a doctor who will accept them as new Medicare patients. As of today, there are about 20 doctors in Anchorage, who are still taking new patients.

Anchorage Neighborhood Center is the only facility still taking new Medicare patients and that facility is being overwhelmed. Providence Family Clinic is no longer taking new patients.

My temporary solution is to offer the names of Nurse Practitioners, who are more than capable of taking care of patients' needs for meds and other physical problems. I have a roster of about 10 PA's, whom I currently recommend.

The problem as I see it, is that doctors charge too much for visits and Medicare pays too little. Obviously Alaska needs more doctors, but it takes almost 10 years for a new doctor to get into business in Alaska. One answer might be for the State of Alaska to offer incentives to outside doctors to come and practice in Alaska. As far as I know, this problem exists in every city in Alaska.

Senator MURKOWSKI. Well, I thank you. Not only for your testimony, Mrs. Hatch, but I thank you for all that you do on behalf of Alaska's seniors. I know that through your efforts, through Older Persons Action Group, you have provided a little bit of comfort as you've tried to help match seniors with providers, and I appreciate that.

I'll come back with questions to each of you, but let's go to you, Mr. Appel. Thank you for being with us this afternoon, and for your work on the Alaska Commission on Aging.

STATEMENT OF FRANK APPEL, CHAIR, ALASKA COMMISSION ON AGING, ANCHORAGE, ALASKA

Mr. APPEL. Senator Murkowski, I'm here to testify on the denial of Medicare services as well, primarily by primary care physicians. I am testifying as an individual who has been denied service, and as Chair of the Alaska Commission on Aging.

Last summer, my primary care physician sent me a letter, stating that he would no longer provide Medicare-reimbursed services. I had been with that physician for about 15 years. The reason stated was that the paperwork was too demanding. He sent along a contract for me to sign, stipulating that I could continue obtaining service, provided I pay for those services personally. I have declined to sign that contract.

I have contacted a few primary care physicians, based on referrals from friends, but I have been unsuccessful in finding a physician. I haven't searched aggressively, because I had a physical last May, however, I do have a prescription that cannot be renewed after April 1st, so I need to get a little bit more aggressive in my effort. My wife has suggested that maybe I need to schedule an appointment for a physical at a clinic in Seattle.

Several weeks ago, a group of us were sitting around the table at a Senior Advocacy Coalition Meeting, the subject was Medicare services, service denials came up. I was astonished when three of the five people who were present, who were over 65, said they had been denied Medicare-reimbursed services, or were unable to find a primary care physician who would accept Medicare patients.

During the last year, the Commission on Aging has received many comments, and much anecdotal evidence that seniors have been denied service, or have been unable to find a primary care physician who will accept new Medicare patients.

They have been told by doctors, if they are not receiving adequate reimbursement to cover their services. Seniors have told us they have made many unsuccessful phone calls to obtain primary care services. I have heard that seniors have increasingly turned to the services of hospital emergency rooms, nurse practitioners, and the neighborhood health clinics.

Recently, I talked to the Executive Director of the Anchorage Neighborhood Health Clinic. She said the Clinic has been overwhelmed recently by the numbers of seniors seeking Medicare and Medicaid services.

Incidentally, most of these comments or complaints have come from the larger communities in this State, the larger population areas. I don't know why that is occurring. I understand there's a shortage of primary care physicians in this State. That shortage may be contributing to the problem.

Under these circumstances, I am concerned that the quality and availability of Medicare medical services for seniors in Alaska is declining, that seniors may have difficulty getting their prescription filled if they cannot find a primary care physician who will sign off on their refill.

Poor or inadequate healthcare may lead to illnesses, and more costly long-term care, and the State and the Federal Government may have to shoulder the burden of these costs. Seniors with resources may decide to move to the Lower 48, where they can obtain medical care, thus removing your economic benefit to the State.

I read a national editorial recently that suggested Medicare reimbursement rates were a form of price control, but that so far, it hasn't reduced the supply of medical services. With the elimination of the Alaskan differential on Medicare reimbursement rates, we may have reached the point where those controlled rates are reducing the supply of services in Alaska.

I think the issue is one of many healthcare-related problems we have facing this Nation. We hear of such large numbers of uninsured citizens. We also read how increasing medical costs are becoming a burden to businesses.

I encourage the Senate to not only address the Medicare issue, but examine some form of comprehensive medical coverage that will deal with our broader healthcare problems. Thank you.

Senator MURKOWSKI. Thank you, Mr. Appel.

And, let's next go to Mr. Carl Berger, the Executive Director at the Lower Kuskokwim Economic Development Council. Welcome, good morning, and your comments, please?

STATEMENT OF CARL BERGER, EXECUTIVE DIRECTOR, LOWER KUSKOKWIM DEVELOPMENT COUNCIL, BETHEL, ALASKA

Mr. BERGER. Thank you, Senator Murkowski. And thank you for the opportunity to speak at this meeting this morning.

I didn't come with any prepared statement, I, in fact, just found out about the location of this hearing about an hour ago. But, I wanted to come because I've recently turned 65, and I had looked forward to getting on to the Medicare program, I'm also a retired State employee, although I continue to work at another job, and I have a good medical coverage plan for working for the State of Alaska, but I don't have a G.P., I don't have a physician. My physician that I have gone to for over 20 years, here in Anchorage, retired, Dr. J. Caldwell. And I have not been able to find anybody else to take his place.

I guess I have to say, lucky for me—I have a heart condition. So, I'm seeing another physician whose specialty is, you know, seeing me for my heart condition. But I'm just baffled by the fact that in this State, you know, what physician in their right mind would want to see me when they can only be reimbursed 40 percent of their usual cost. That's just, you know, it doesn't jive at all with the way things should be.

I was pleased to see that there was a program in place, up until the beginning of this year, I believe, or last year, to allow for better reimbursement to physicians. I pointed this out in a letter to you and to the other members of the congressional delegation, that we must do something about this. I'm not speaking only for myself, I'm actually in pretty good shape, I do have medical insurance, but there are other people in the bush who do not.

It's difficult to find a physician, even at the Yukon-Kuskokwim Health Corporation, because they are fully booked, as well. And as a non-Native person, I'm not really eligible to be seen there, except as an emergency situation. So I don't think that's the solution, either. I'm willing to pay my way into Anchorage to see a physician. But right now, I can't find one, and that's wrong, that needs to be fixed. Not just for me, but for a lot of other people around the State.

So, I guess I'll leave my comments at that, and be happy to answer any questions you may have. Thank you for the opportunity to speak.

Senator MURKOWSKI. Thank you. I appreciate the comments from all three of you.

It's one thing to have statistics, it's another thing to have the real stories on the ground. And whether they're as unscientific as a group of folks sitting around a kitchen table talking about what has happened, in terms of denial to access—these are real-live stories, these are Alaskans that do not have access. And, it makes our statistics all that more compelling.

Mrs. Hatch, let me ask you—you'd indicated that you kind of conducted a telephone survey of the facilities in Anchorage to kind of determine who was accepting new Medicare patients. How long ago was this? Or, are you still doing it now?

Ms. HATCH. This is ongoing.

Senator MURKOWSKI. You're still doing it now. And, that's how you have come to your number of——

Ms. HATCH. Well, there's three questions we ask. We ask, Are you taking new Medicare patients now? Are you taking new Medicare patients? Do you take assignment of Medicare? And we generally try to get the billing person, or whoever's in charge of the bills in the office. And we can call at 1 a.m., and they say, "yes, they are taking new Medicare patients," and you can call them back in the afternoon to get another telephone number, or an address, and they say, "no, we're not taking them." So, it's incredible.

Senator MURKOWSKI. And, as you're kind of acting as a facilitator for some of the seniors that you're working with, you've suggested that if they can't get into a practitioner, that a nurse practitioner is the next best option. But, what happens if their medical needs go beyond what a nurse practitioner can provide?

Ms. HATCH. Nurse practitioners usually work with a doctor, and they can usually get them in to see a doctor.

Senator MURKOWSKI. So, we're not seeing the same wall, then?

Ms. HATCH. There's not the same wall. Because if a nurse practitioner asks you to, you know, refers you to a doctor, they'll generally take them.

And that's the same with specialists, too. If a doctor refers you to a specialist, that specialist will generally take you.

Senator MURKOWSKI. Right.

Ms. HATCH. As a Medicare patient.

Senator MURKOWSKI. Mr. Appel, you've mentioned that you have—through the Commission—been in conversation with many seniors that are focused, and very concerned, on this same issue. Is it fair to say that the situation that we're seeing here in Anchorage is replicated around the State? Or, do you have conversations with folks outside the Anchorage area?

Mr. APPEL. Well, we've had conversations with people in some of the smaller communities of this State—Ketchikan, Juneau, specifically—because we've held meetings there recently. And, it doesn't appear to be as much of an issue in those communities. And I can't speculate why that is, but it could be that those communities are more insular or more intimate, and so physicians may be reluctant to refuse services in a smaller community.

But, most of our comments come from the Rail Belt area—the Matsu, Anchorage, and Fairbanks—the larger population areas. But, we have not explored this issue in the rural community, so I would hesitate to comment and say——

Senator MURKOWSKI. Does the Commission on Aging do a similar thing that Mrs. Hatch has described, in terms of trying to do an assessment of who is available to take new Medicare patients? Are you involved in that at all?

Mr. APPEL. Well, we examined some of the State organizations. At a meeting we had in November, one of the Medicare-coordinating agencies for the State suggested they had a list of physicians that accepted Medicare, but we found out that that was not the case. And so we couldn't—because we wanted to advise seniors where they could obtain services. So, we have been unsuccessful in finding any kind of a list, or any kind of a method of identifying physicians who take Medicare.

Senator MURKOWSKI. Mrs. Hatch, do you want to weigh in on that?

Ms. HATCH. Just another——

Senator MURKOWSKI. If you can put the microphone——

Ms. HATCH [continuing]. That list that Frank is talking about, it's on the Medicare web page. And it's doctors who have taken Medicare, or are enrolled in Medicare. But that doesn't mean they're taking new Medicare patients. So, the list is really worthless.

Also, I don't know if you've had anything to do in Fairbanks, but I've gotten reports in Fairbanks that doctors are asking for a $300 "retainer," just to take you on as a Medicare patient.

Senator MURKOWSKI. Well, I had a series of Town Hall Meetings last year on this issue of the physician shortage—one up in Fairbanks, one on the Kenai Peninsula, and one down in Juneau—and heard very similar comments and concerns about the access issue.

Mr. Berger, from the Bethel area—you've pointed out that your situation might, perhaps, be a little bit different, but in terms of access in the more rural parts of this State, I'm assuming that you're not an isolated instance, that many are faced with the same issues that you have described here this morning.

Mr. BERGER. I think they are. One thing I didn't mention in my earlier comments was the importance of the continuity of care. Having a general practitioner for almost 25 years before he retired was important to me. I worked hard to get my medical coverage with the State of Alaska, it's good coverage. But, it's not much use to me if I can't find somebody who will see me on a regular basis. I don't want to have to skip around, from one doctor to a nurse practitioner, to a physician's assistant. I want to establish a relationship with a doctor that I can see on a regular basis. And if he's in Anchorage, so be it. If he's somewhere else, that's fine.

But I don't want to have to be forced to go from one person to another who doesn't really know me, and never really does get to know me and my medical situation. I think that's very important. And, as somebody who has established a career, and is now getting ready to retire—having just turned 65—I'd like to look forward to having good, reliable, steady care from a person, a physician, that I can get to know and feel comfortable with, and who will take better care of me than somebody who sees me once and never sees me again. Or, maybe twice, or three times, and then I'm jumped to somebody else, and then somebody else after that. And I think there are other people in the bush that are in that same situation that I am in.

Senator MURKOWSKI. I'm going to ask one last question of all of you, and it will be the same question.

Given the array of issues and concerns that face us in Alaska and in the Nation regarding healthcare, what is the biggest problem? What's the biggest problem—is it access? Is it the cost? Very briefly—what's the biggest problem with healthcare from your perspective?

Mrs. Hatch, if you can speak into the microphone.

Ms. HATCH. Access to doctors, I think, is the most important thing. Because if you can't find a doctor, what are you going to do?

Senator MURKOWSKI. Right. Thank you.

Mr. Appel.

Mr. APPEL. Well, I think, certainly access to doctors by seniors over 65 is a huge problem, but I think medical costs, in general, having been spiraling, and so I see that as a problem as well.

Senator MURKOWSKI. Mr. Berger.

Mr. BERGER. I think it's access to physicians, but I also think the insurance companies who provide coverage to Alaskans, need to have a better understanding of the cost of care here, and that it's higher. I often get my charges rejected, because they're above the usual customary charges. And then I ask my doctor—the heart doctor that I can see—he says, "Oh no, there's nobody in Alaska who will provide this service at the rate they're willing to reimburse." And that kind of makes me angry, you know, I pay for my health insurance through my employment, and so I've challenged the insurance company to say, "Wait a minute, your usual and customary charge isn't really the usual and customary charge in Alaska," and you know what? They back right down. And so far I've had pretty good results on getting them to reconsider and pay.

But that shouldn't be necessary. Insurance companies that are based in Seattle or somewhere else should be willing to pay what physicians charge here, or what a service like an echocardiogram costs in this State. Yes, you can get an echocardiogram done in Seattle, but do they really want to fly me down there? Oh, no, they surely do not. But they want to pay for what an echocardiogram costs in Seattle, not what it costs in Anchorage, or somewhere else here in Alaska. So, that needs to be addressed, too. Thank you.

Senator MURKOWSKI. Very good. I appreciate again the testimony, the perspective that you bring, and all that you are doing individually, collectively, to help make a difference. As you point out, we've got some real problems when it comes to access, when it comes to costs, and how we explain our higher costs in the State. So, thank you for what you're doing, we'll keep working on it as well. Thank you for serving on the panel.

And with that, we will bring the next panel forward, and this is the panel that has been asked to speak to the potential solutions to the patient access crisis.

Having heard from users within the system about the problems that we face, we now want to hear from some who would offer some suggestions.

We will have Dr. Ross Tanner, Dr. Harold Johnston, Dr. Richard Neubauer, Dr. Byron Perkins, Dr. John Coombs and Ms. Karen Perdue join us at the table.

And for the audience, I'll give a little bit of background on each of our panelists this morning. Dr. Ross Tanner is the President-Elect of the Alaska State Medical Association; Dr. Harold Johnston is the Director of the Alaska Family Practice Residency program; Dr. Richard Neubauer here in Anchorage is a doctor in internal medicine; we have Dr. Byron Perkins, who is the President of the Alaska Osteopathic Association; we have Dr. John Coombs, who is the Associate Vice-President for Medical Affairs, and the Dean for Graduate Medical Programs there, the WWAMI program; and we have Karen Perdue, Associate Vice-President for Health at the University of Alaska, and the one who will explain to us the details and the findings from the Alaska Physicians Supply Task Force.

So with that, if we can move from you, Dr. Tanner, on down the line and I will reserve my questions until all of you have had an opportunity to present.

So, thank you for being here.

Dr. Tanner.

STATEMENT OF ROSS TANNER, PRESIDENT-ELECT, ALASKA STATE MEDICAL ASSOCIATION, ANCHORAGE, ALASKA

Dr. TANNER. Good morning, Senator.

Senator MURKOWSKI. Good morning.

I'm going to ask everyone to make sure that that mike is pulled pretty close up. I understand it's been tough for some of the folks in the back to hear. So——

Dr. TANNER. As the first physician to testify, I'd like to request Secret Service agents to protect my well-being before I leave here today.

[Laughter.]

But I am the President-Elect of the Alaska State Medical Association, and as many of you know, the Alaska State Medical Association, or ASMA, represents physicians statewide, and is primarily concerned with the healthcare of all Alaskans, and that's all Alaskans—young, old, and middle-aged. And I don't know how to define old age, other than saying Medicare-age.

ASMA is also federated with the American Medical Association. Welcome back to Alaska, it's nice to see you again, and thank you for the opportunity to address you today. It is, indeed, an honor to be able to address the Senate Committee on Health, Education, Labor, and Pensions.

Last week, I participated and represented the State of Alaska at the AMA National Advocacy Conference in Washington, DC., which addressed many of the concerns which we will discuss here today.

As President, I receive no remuneration for my services, or the time away from my busy medical practice. So, why would anybody want to become involved in organized medicine?

It is the progressive deterioration of access, as well as inefficiency of delivery of healthcare to the citizens of this State, and also of people of other States, that—in the last 15 years, I believe that this is continuing to worsen, and I believe the prognosis is poor. This is shameful, given our intellectual and financial resources we have as a Nation.

Today, I would like to provide you with a current assessment regarding Alaska's chronic, and currently acute, shortage of physicians, and to provide you with ASMA's recommendations on how you can help us address this critical situation that endangers the healthcare of every Alaskan.

Currently, Alaska has a shortage of 30 percent of physicians, or nearly 400 physicians. Alaska has 10 slots per year at the University of Washington Medical School program, participation with the collaborative effort between the five States, the WWAMI program, which is Washington, Wyoming, Alaska, Montana and Idaho.

Alaska has only one residency program, the Alaska Family Medicine Residency, which would train a maximum of 12 residents per year. Alaska has a physician workforce that has more age than most other States, and over the next 20 years, Alaska will need to nearly double the number of physicians, just to keep pace with the expected population growth. This requires a net increase of 50 physicians per year, given the projection of the number of physicians who will leave practice, which will require approximately 100 physicians per year to be added to the workforce currently.

Alaska has experienced a large number of retired military, Medicare-eligible people, seeking treatment by private physicians due to the deployment of Alaskan military physicians to the Middle East. These numbers were developed by the Alaska Physicians Supply Task Force that we heard about earlier. This Task Force was convened by the University of Alaska President, Mark Hamilton, and Alaska State Commissioner of the Department of Health and Social Services, Karleen Jackson.

The Task Force reported their findings after working for at least 6 months in its report, "Securing an Adequate Number of Physicians for Alaska's Needs." ASMA was represented on this Task Force by our Executive Director, Mr. Jim Jordan, who is with us today, and I believe that you all have been provided with this report.

For Senators and people of this committee that come from larger States, some of these issues may not seem that large, at face. However, when put in perspective to other States, the Alaska picture is, indeed, grim. Alaska has the sixth lowest physician to population ration in the Nation, as you earlier stated. Most physicians practice within 100 miles of where they will complete their residency or specialty training.

Alaska has only one residency program with 12 slots of family medicine residents. By contrast, as reported by the Texas Medical Association, Texas has nearly 6,400 resident slots in multiple specialties. New York has over 15,000 slots, California has nearly 9,000 slots, and Pennsylvania has almost 7,000 slots—just for residencies. If 12 slots were sufficient for Alaska's roughly 650,000 population, that would mean in comparison, that Texas' 6,400 slots would be adequate for a population of 325 million people—very much underserved.

Alaska has only 10 slots at the University of Washington Medical School, coupled with the 12 family medicine residency slots, cannot come anywhere near the growing need that our public and our citizens of this State need. Alaska's current physician workforce is not sufficient to provide the clinical teaching resources necessary to expand the residency program itself, for a wide variety of needed specialists.

An increase in the WWAMI Program, or additional slots through other medical schools, will not provide any help for a minimum of 10 years, because of the duration of medical training that all of us went through that are sitting at this table.

Recruitment costs in Alaska range anywhere from $60,000 to upward to $200,000 per physician. I think you will agree that the current physician workforce environment in Alaska is in a crisis, as we've heard from patients, as well as you're hearing from physicians today. This is particularly true when taken in the context that Alaska needs to recruit physicians from other parts of the country at a time when there is also a nationwide shortage of physicians, and it's projected to be between 80,000 to 200,000 physicians—truly, alarmingly large numbers.

Before I outline what ASMA recommends for ways in which you can help Alaskans get the healthcare they need and deserve, I would like to briefly describe what we are doing at a State level.

For the past 10 years, ASMA has been instrumental in advocating for legislation that would create and maintain an environment conducive to attracting, and most importantly, retaining physicians. Those successful measures include major liability reform in 1997, and again in 2005—and I want to thank you for that—enacting an Alaska Bill of Rights, protecting patients, enacting fair contracting provisions for relationships between physicians and health insurers, enacting Health Insurance Prompt Payment Law, and enacting legislation that allows physicians to jointly negotiate with insurers for everything but their fees.

These measures, as well as others, were critical for my decision to come to Alaska. If you think it's bad in Alaska, go to Washington State—it's worse. Since I've last left the area around Olympia, there's been 40 physicians leave since I've been here, for 2 years, just in that one community. And before I got there, there were 50 physicians left in the preceding year. It's worse.

Currently, ASMA—along with other key organizations, such as the Hospital and Nursing Home Association, and the University of Alaska—is acting as the catalyst to enact a bill to double the WWAMI class size from 10 to 20 medical students. The State legislature is expected to act on the bill in early 2007, so that in the fall, a total of 20 qualified Alaskans can enter medical school at the University of Washington.

ASMA is also exploring ways to develop long-term, sustainable funding mechanism for physician education for qualified Alaskans.

Here's what I think you can do too at the national level to help Alaska—and patients in Alaska—and really, across the Nation. No. 1, enact a legislation that permanently, and I stress, permanently, fixes the Medicare physician payment system so that it realistically reflects the physician practice cost. With rising costs, coupled with shrinking reimbursements, this leaves less quality time with your doctor, if you even get it.

In general, I will need to see approximately 45 Medicare patients in a day, that produces about the same revenue as 20 insured patients to equal each other. As an internist, I lack the ability to generate revenue by procedures, and am compensated for cognitive and diagnostic abilities.

No. 2, if a patient is new to Alaska, or my patients turn 65 years of age, it will be nearly impossible to find a primary care physician, as we've heard today, eloquently placed by patients and our Commissioner. My own mother and father encountered this problem. It is certainly nobody's fault for turning 65 years of age.

Alaska reportedly has the second-fastest growing elderly population, second only to Nevada. Continued year to year, uncertainty created by the flawed sustainable growth rate, or SGR formulate, has caused a lack of access to care for Alaska Medicare beneficiaries. Medicare payments to physicians in Alaska represent 37 to 40 percent of the cost of opening our doors each day.

No. 3, we ask that you support and enact legislation that provides tax credits for young physicians to practice in frontier States, such as Alaska. Your bill, S. 290, is such a bill. This will help Alaska, and other frontier and rural States, to attract physicians.

No. 4, support and enact legislation that revamps the funding of graduate medical education. Reforms need to be made that recognize residencies, like the family practice residency, in Alaska, and make them eligible for Federal funding support, as well as other mechanisms that would encourage regional residencies between States such as Alaska, Wyoming, Montana and Washington State. Furthermore, the latitude to work with Canada is needed. Alaska could work in conjunction with Canadian medical schools, or with residencies in Western and Northwestern Canada to develop joint residencies.

No. 5, develop programs to help medical students cope with the enormous debt of going to medical school. Our best and brightest students are being disincentivized from going to medical school due to the tremendous educational debt associated with medical training. For public medical schools, it is an average of $125,000 per student, and for private medical schools, it is approximately $200,000 to go to school. For those bright students not deterred by the debt, it is impacting their choice of specialty training. Many physicians are choosing their career path, based on potential future income.

So, now students are often going into more lucrative sub-specialties, than going into family practice or general internal medicine. A way to remove these disincentives must be found.

Others here today will speak to many of these same issues that I've mentioned, such as Dr. Johnson, on graduate medical education, Dr. Neubauer on the practice of internal medicine, Dr. Perkins with primary care and family practice, and I hope the testimony today by myself, and others, does not fall on deaf ears.

I would also imagine that it is a rare occasion when a specific occupation, business, or trade comes and asks you to increase competition. And, as I stated in the beginning, the physicians are genuinely concerned with the healthcare of all Alaskans.

I'd be happy to address any questions you may have. Thank you.

Senator MURKOWSKI. Thank you, Dr. Tanner.

Dr. Johnston.

STATEMENT OF HAROLD JOHNSTON, DIRECTOR, ALASKA FAMILY PRACTICE RESIDENCY, ANCHORAGE, ALASKA

Dr. JOHNSTON. Thank you, Senator. It's a great pleasure to be able to offer testimony to the committee. And I congratulate you on all of the work that you've done to help us so far, here in Alaska, with our healthcare crisis issues.

I'm the Director of the Alaska Family Medicine Residency, the only graduate medical education program in Alaska, and I also have had the distinct privilege to be the co-chair of the Alaska Physician Supply Task Force, whose report has been cited several times so far today.

I appreciate the remarks of Dr. Tanner, much of what he said were things that I had intended to say, as well, so I'm not going to repeat those. But, I want to emphasize a couple of points about things that he said.

One, about physician education in Alaska—indeed, Alaska has the lowest, per capita number of medical school slots in the United States, we have the lowest number of residency slots in the United States, we have the lowest acceptance rate of Alaskan medical students, Alaska students into medical school, of any population in the United States. And, the fact that we are so far behind is contributing to our crisis——

Senator MURKOWSKI. Can you repeat that last one? We have the lowest number of——

Dr. JOHNSTON. We have the lowest——

Senator MURKOWSKI [continuing]. Number of students being accepted into medical schools?

Dr. JOHNSTON. We have the lowest acceptance rate of students going into medical schools. In other words, of all of the Alaska students who apply to medical school, we have the lowest rate of acceptance.

Senator MURKOWSKI. Thank you.

Dr. JOHNSTON. Those facts are contributing greatly to the crisis that we have in physician supply here. As has been stated, rural areas are in tremendous shortage. In rural areas, and nonrural areas, we have a lot of specialties that are in shortage, primary care is in major crisis, particularly in Anchorage, general internal medicine is in extreme and dire shortage, although many specialties are in shortage here, as well.

I believe that these problems are related to the consequences of national trends. Many of those national trends are things that can be affected by Congress, especially in the Medicare program, but also in other ways.

One of the national trends is the national shortage. Years ago, in the 1980s, multiple specialties societies, and the Council on Graduate Medical Education—using flawed methodology—concluded there would be a surplus of physicians. As a consequence of that analysis, the Association of American Medical Colleges reduced the number of medical student slots that they were producing—or reduced their growth rate, anyway, and Congress in 1997, capped the number of residency positions that were available for funding in the United States.

About a year after Congress capped the number of residency positions, the light started to dawn that the analysis had been flawed, and actually, in 2005 COGME reversed its position, and stated that its previous analysis was wrong, and that actually we were facing a shortage of physicians, and that the caps were a mistake. The Association of American Medical Colleges around the same time, advocated an increase of medical student positions of 30 percent over what currently exists in the United States, in order to start the valve—open the valve on the pipeline of physician production.

Well, in Alaska, we have always been a net importer of physicians. We don't have much training capacity, as I stated before, and so in order to supply ourselves with physicians, we have had to recruit them from the Lower 48. Well, when the Lower 48 has a shortage of physicians, that makes the recruitment to Alaska increasingly difficult, and part of the reason that we're seeing the cost of recruitment go up, and the cost of absent physicians go up so high across the State, is because it is becoming more and more difficult to get doctors in here. It used to be that the Indian Health Service would assign commissioned officers to Alaska, and the military had a different process of assigning physicians to Alaska—many of Alaska's physicians came from doctors who were in the commissioned corps of the military, and then in their assigned rotation, here, fell in love with Alaska and decided to stay after their obligations expired.

Currently, that process is no longer effective in Alaska, because the presence of the Indian Health Service in the commissioned corps, and the military, has been reduced. The commissioned corps has been reduced, the military has changed its policies, and so the assignments are in a different mechanism that I don't fully understand, but it effects the ability of military physicians to enter private practice in Alaska.

So, on one hand, the recruitment problem is partly due to the national shortage. That can be traced back to the training limitations that have been posed by Congress.

Second, primary care shortage is due partly to the general physician shortage, but also to a great degree to the problem of getting doctors to go into primary care. Student debt is very high, graduating from medical school. And nonprimary care specialties pay much better than primary care. Students are responsive, to some degree, to the financial incentives that they experience as they enter practice. And the effect of that has been to diminish the interest in primary care by graduating medical students.

Part of the reason is the debt—part of the reason is that payments to primary care doctors are lower than payments to nonprimary care doctors. The testimony earlier today from people who have been trying to get Medicare patients into doctors has stated that they don't have much trouble getting patients into specialists. But they have a terrible time getting patients into primary care doctors. As a practicing physician, that's my experience, as well. When I have—as a primary care doctor—made a diagnosis, and advised the patient to seek surgery, or a specialty services, I can refer them to one of my specialty colleagues, and unfailingly get that patient in to be seen. But, getting the patient in the door of the primary care office is the big, big problem.

One big problem for Alaska, now, is related to these caps on residencies. We know what works. Our family medicine residency program has been a stunning success. We graduate 12 residents per year—we will be graduating 12, we're in the growth phase now, right now we're graduating 10 per year—but in another 2 years, we'll be graduating 12 per year. Seventy-five percent of our graduates practice in Alaska. Fifty-five percent of them practice in a rural community. If you count Alaska practice, rural practice, or underserved practice—such as an Indian health service, or community health center as a target—95 percent of our graduates practice in one of the socially desirable target practices. We know how to do it. And we're doing a good job of it. But, we can't do enough, because they have caps. Our residency program, in 2 years, we'll be training 36 residents at a time, but our cap for Federal payment is at 22. We can't get that cap lifted, and consequently, the program is running at a very large deficit, which has been sustained by the private business that sponsors it, not by the government or the society as a whole.

We also need lots more residencies in Alaska. Family medicine is not the only specialty we need. We desperately need residencies in several other specialties which could easily be started in Alaska. There are plenty of talented doctors to teach, and plenty of interesting patient cases to learn from. I think our experience in the family medicine program indicates we could be very successful in recruiting students from other schools to come to Alaska to train, but none of these programs can start in this State, because there's no Federal money to pay for the resident FTEs.

Most of the other specialties, besides family medicine, can only be well-trained in a large community, like Anchorage. And, hospitals in large communities like Anchorage are capped. So, we need to have relief of these resident FTE caps, in order to initiate a funding stream that can start training programs for the other doctors.

I think that as we look into the future of physician shortages in Alaska, we have to move forward on all fronts—the Physician Supply Task Force identifies a number of them, and Dr. Tanner has identified most of them in his comments. We have to move forward on the front of retention so that we can keep the doctors we have practicing longer, and happier, we need to move forward on the front of recruitment, because that's the short-term way of getting doctors into the State—if we start recruitment efforts now, we'll be able to get doctors soon.

But, those two efforts are not going to be enough, in the long run. We have to also start training our own doctors in much larger numbers, because as the competition for physicians gets tighter and tighter around the United States, unless we're training our own, we are always going to be unable to attract the doctors that we need for this State.

With that, I'll conclude my testimony, and answer your questions.

Senator MURKOWSKI. Very interesting comments, thank you, Dr. Johnston.

And next, let's go to Dr. Richard Neubauer. Welcome, and good morning.

STATEMENT OF RICHARD NEUBAUER, INTERNAL MEDICINE, ANCHORAGE, ALASKA

Dr. NEUBAUER. I'm very pleased to give this testimony.

Besides being a general internist here in Anchorage, I also serve on the Board of Regents for the American College of Physicians, which is the second-largest physician group in the country, representing about 120,000 general internists, and other internists. Second only to the American Medical Association.

As I listen this morning, it struck me that one thing that hasn't been said is how much joy there is in being a doctor. You know, I really love my job, I enjoy being a general internist, it's a wonderful job—perhaps the best job in medicine. And it's a real tragedy that we have to be here talking about the delivery of medical care, or the lack of access to medical care, in the way we are.

So, just prefacing my remarks, I think that this is very, very important.

While there are shortages in many specialties in medicine, it's the shortage of primary care physicians—and, specifically, general internists—that concerns me the most. In my view, these areas of medicine are actually near collapse, both here and nationally. And are critically threatened, unless there are prompt actions that are taken to reverse these current trends.

When I graduated from medical school at Yale University in 1976, and then did my internship and residency at the University of Michigan from 1976 to 1979, the majority of my classmates wanted to be internists of one sort or another.

Nowadays, that's very different. And, the majority of medical school graduates want to pursue careers in radiology, ophthalmology, anesthesia or dermatology, because these areas of medicine have a kindlier lifestyle, better pay, and are perceived to have better prestige than what I do right now. This is especially tragic, I think, because with an increasing elderly population, the need for general internists who are skilled in the management of complex medical problems is increasing, and will continue to increase. And, I think the testimony that's been given earlier today testifies to that, as well.

After leaving my residency training and completing a scholarship obligation with the Indian Health Service in Wyoming, I came to Alaska in 1981, and have been in practice here since. When I started my career, I typically cared for 10 or 15 hospitalized patients, took many admissions from the emergency room, and worked, as well, full-time in my office, and didn't get home until really late at night.

Over 25 years of practice, I've watched as many of my colleagues in internal medicine have retired, moved away, or moved on to other things. With very few exceptions, as these physicians have left their practices, they have been unable to find young physicians to take their place, and have simply closed their doors. And, with that, their patients have been scattered to the wind, hopefully to find other doctors, oftentimes not being able to.

And, nowadays, when this happens here in Anchorage—especially if these patients are covered by Medicare, they can't find doctors to care for them.

An example of that was, a physician in my office who retired earlier this year, and we've literally had patients coming to the front desk in tears, trying to find a physician to care for them. And we try to help with that, as much as we can, but it's very limited, given limited manpower capabilities.

The reason for this is because these patients have very complex problems, that take a lot of time to take care of properly. And frankly, the reimbursement for seeing them does not even cover the overhead of operating an office.

So, as has been said by others, these patients are destined to use the emergency room for their primary care, and that's both inexpensive and inefficient. And, oftentimes, these patients may also neglect their problems until they become more far advanced, and are thus either harder, or impossible, to treat.

Right now, unfortunately, there's virtually no financial incentive for a young primary care physician, in internal medicine, to come start a private practice in this city. The remuneration for their efforts would simply not be enough to justify the work involved, and the overhead of operating an office.

Starting in the mid-1990s, in Anchorage and elsewhere, there was an advent of a new area of medicine called "hospitalice medicine," this is internists who only work in the hospital, and this even further changed the dynamics of care in Anchorage, and around the country.

Right now, in general, internists who are coming out of training programs are only interested in getting hospitalice, and not operating in an office. This is, again, due to the high overhead of office practice, the burden of unreimbursed work in an office, and the threat of punitive audits, the long hours, constant need to be on-call, and low compensation, in general, for the work in our current reimbursement system.

With the ascendancy of hospitalice practice, this has certainly benefited functionality of inpatient care, but it has, unfortunately, come at the expense of promoting a further decline—critical decline—in the interest of providing long-term management in ambulatory or outpatient settings.

Right now, in Anchorage, by my count—and I could be off a little bit on this—there are about 18 general internists working in office settings, and by comparison, there are approximately 30 cardiologists in Anchorage. And this is just not a healthy mix.

A sad truth is that if I—at age 57, not quite 65, but getting there—were to become incapacitated, or otherwise leave my practice, it's highly unlikely that anyone would be around to take my place, and my patients would be without a physician.

Let me just present an example from my own practice of how coordination of care of a patient by primary care physicians can result in better outcomes, and lower costs, but is actually not reimbursed by the current system.

I currently care for a man in his fifties who, tragically, has had a series of strokes and heart attacks at a very young age. He suffers with congestive heart failure, but with modern medical management, has lived with these conditions for a number of years, whereas in the past, he probably would have been dead by now. He also has diabetes, hypertension, many psychological issues that have complicated his care. And I share his care with a cardiologist, but for quite some time, he was visiting the emergency room on a regular basis with chest pain, was often admitted to the hospital at great cost, and with no particular benefit to his care.

By intervening and allowing him open telephone access to my nursing staff, to the physician assistant, who I recently hired to help me, and having him come to my office for frequent reviews of his medications with my staff, we've been actually able to avert most of his emergency room visits.

This was done with low-cost office visits, unreimbursed time in person and on the telephone with him, and the monetary savings to the system were tremendous. Whereas the monetary benefit to my office was modest.

What can be done about these problems? I think both here and in Alaska and nationwide, a further study of the manpower needs for primary care services is sorely needed. In my view, the current methods that CMS uses to track access to care are very blunt tools that, just frankly, don't reflect reality. It's my view that a robust, primary care presence in our country will require a restructuring of the payment systems in a way that reflects the importance of primary care services, with recognition that much of what we currently do is unreimbursed.

I think management fees, above and beyond traditional fee-for-service reimbursement, would be one step, at least, in recognizing the value of primary care of the patient, and needs to be strongly considered.

I think new models of care, such as the advanced medical home concept proposed by the American College of Physicians, has promised to increase the attractiveness of internal medicine as a career. This model relies heavily on electronic medical records to improve the functionality and accountability of practices, and to improve the delivery of preventive services, but the implementation of this technology, namely electronic health records, has been hampered by high cost, and difficulty of deployment in busy offices.

We do have an HER, Electronic Health Record alliance here, that has been formed by the APS, the Alaska Physicians and Surgeons, the Alaska Chapter of the American College of Physicians, and the State Medical Association to try and address this, and we're trying to get funding for a pilot program here to see how we could implement these records better.

I think medical training programs need to be re-designed to encourage students to consider careers in internal medicine, and primary care, but that has not been happening in a concerted fashion, partly due to entrenched interests, and perverse incentives. And this certainly needs to change.

As has been said, students are burdened with so much debt coming out of medical training, that they're pushed into higher paid specialties by necessity. In an effort to fill positions that graduates of American medical schools are not interested in, as a Nation, we've been robbing other countries of their own talented physicians, but importing foreign graduates, and this is certainly not a good, long-term global strategy.

In summary, I think we stand at a critical time in the design of delivery systems within our medical communities. Certainly, inaction at this time will have very predictable results. A lopsided supply of physicians in very high paid specialties, coupled with access to care problems for patients who want the guidance of a physician to coordinate their medical care.

There are things we can do to positively shape the future, but this will require, I think, courage and conviction, and I certainly applaud your efforts in this regard.

I'll conclude by asking that the HELP committee require a study and report on ways that the Federal Government can increase the attractiveness of primary care, including consideration of programs to eliminate or reduce student debt, for those who go into primary care, redesigning Federal support for medical education, to expose medical students to well-functioning models of community-based primary care, and changes in Federal reimbursement policies to support the value of primary care.

Thank you very much.

Senator MURKOWSKI. Thank you, Dr. Neubauer. I appreciate your testimony.

And, let's move over to the other table here, we have Dr. Byron Perkins, the President of the Alaska—I was going to say, it's not the American Osteopathic Association, you're the Alaska rep for the American Osteopath.

STATEMENT OF BYRON PERKINS, AMERICAN OSTEOPATIC ASSOCIATION, PRESIDENT OF THE ALASKA OSTEOPATHIC MEDICAL ASSOCIATION, ANCHORAGE, ALASKA

Dr. PERKINS. That's correct. Thank you, Senator Murkowski.

Senator MURKOWSKI. Thank you, and welcome.

Dr. PERKINS. I am Byron Perkins, and I am a practicing osteopathic family physician here in Anchorage, and I am the President of the Alaska Osteopathic Medical Association, AKOMA.

I've had the privilege of working in Alaska 4 years in Nome, and 7 years with the Alaskan Native Medical Center, and now in primary care/private practice in Anchorage.

I'm honored to be here today representing the American Osteopathic Association, and AKOMA. The AOA represents the Nation's 59,000 osteopathic physicians, and over 12,000 osteopathic medical students, and we applaud your interest in this very timely discussion, and important issue.

Much of my testimony will echo the findings of the Alaska Physician Supply Task Force Committee. We applaud their work, we were able to participate in testimony on their efforts. Much of my testimony will echo some of the testimony already presented.

The AOA recognizes that many communities in the United States face limited access to physicians, and physician services. We've heard that today, this is especially true in rural and frontier communities, and really so in Alaska. And for more than 130 years, AOA has been dedicated to training and educating the future physician workforce. We have a tradition of turning out primary care physicians. More than 65 percent of our students, physician graduates, practice in primary care, and that trend has been historical.

In Alaska, there are 115 licensed osteopathic physicians, 77 of those physicians practice in primary care, roughly 69 percent. They practice in diverse communities, from places like Barrow, and Bethel and Craig and Klowak, Nome, Gotsebu, and Anchorage/ Fairbanks, Juneau.

Over the past 15 years, the osteopathic profession has enjoyed tremendous growth. We are currently one of the fastest-growing professions in healthcare. Since 1990, the osteopathic physician numbers have increased 67 percent, there are currently about 59,000 osteopathic physicians in the United States, we are still a minority in physician groups. About 6 percent of all physicians in the United States are osteopathic physicians.

As our membership grows, the AOA is refocusing our efforts on our core mission, which is training physicians who are capable and willing to provide high-quality care to our Nation's neediest populations, particularly in primary care.

Many experts believe that we are in a shortfall, we in Alaska have made the same conclusion—we are in a physician shortage. If we begin to work on that effort now, we can make a difference, as we begin to educate and train a larger number of physicians in the immediate near future.

The time it takes to educate and train a physician is anywhere from 7 to 14 years, and that means anybody starting in school today won't be available to serve for at least 7 years, particularly in primary care. And due to the time education requirements for future physicians, we believe a concerted effort must be made now, and that is what most of my testimony is referencing today.

Today, one in five medical students in the United States is in osteopathic medical school. Currently, there are 23 colleges of osteopathic medicine, operating on 26 campuses. There are two additional colleges that will open within the next 2 years, bringing the total number of colleges to 25, operating on 28 campuses. In 2007, those colleges will graduate approximately 3,000 new physicians, by 2008, approximately 3,500 physicians, and by the year 2015, we are projecting 5,000 new physicians per year.

We, in Alaska, are especially proud of the Pacific-Northwest University of Health Sciences, projected to open in the year 2008 in Yakima, Washington. This has been a collaborative effort, and by the five Northwestern States, and the associations in those States, we believe the opportunity to participate in this will give us more direct influence on the number of students, and the type of students that will be referring and matriculating to this facility. I'm optimistic that when it begins operating, it will be a direct contributing factor to Alaska's physician workforce, in the future. And that recommendation did come forward in the Physician Supply Task Force recommendations.

Medical schools, and colleges of osteopathic medicine traditionally place significant emphasis on an applicant's academic achievement. We agree with this, but we also believe that medical school should be looking at the whole person, that is something that is traditionally done in the osteopathic applications process. Particularly, when a student from Alaska, or from a rural community, is evaluated—they should meet all of those academic requirements, but at the same time, there is something desirable about placing a student from a rural community into a medical school.

If two students are equally qualified, we would encourage schools to matriculate students from the rural communities. Much of the same testimony has come forward.

Additionally, our medical education system must increase its efforts to promote both primary care specialties, and experience in rural practice locations. It's already been testified to by Dr. Johnston and Dr. Neubauer. The role of the family physician and the internal medicine physician generalist is less glamorous, less rewarding financially, and yet I would echo what Dr. Neubauer said, this is the greatest thing in the world to do. I love my work, I wouldn't trade it for anything, I am blessed to be an osteopathic physician.

The issues facing our Nation's rural healthcare system are complex, and there are no easy answers. The AOA recommends five policy changes that we believe will lead to improved access to physician services, and increase the availability of U.S.-trained physicians. And, I would like to list those now.

No. 1, the Congress should consider eliminating the cap on available, and funded, residency positions in the United States. Dr. Johnston spoke to this, there are currently, approximately 96,000 funded residency positions. The number of funded residency positions has been static since the 1990s, when the Balanced Budget Act of 1997 put a cap on residency positions. This severely limits our ability to increase the residency positions available here, in Alaska—not just Alaska, all of the Pacific Northwest.

The AOA encourages Congress to either remove or increase the caps on the number of funded, graduate medical education training slots, as established by the Budget Act of 1997. This past week, legislations were introduced in the Senate that would accomplish this goal. The Resident Physicians Shortage Reduction Act of 2007, increases the cap adjustments for teaching hospitals in eligible States, where there is a demonstrated shortage of resident positions. Alaska is 1 of 24 States that would benefit from this legislation, and AOA supports this legislation, and urges all Senators to go sponsor this important bill.

We would, in that vein, support the Physician Shortage Elimination Act that you referenced in your opening statement. I think it's the right direction to move.

No. 2, in addition to expanding the training capacity at existing teaching hospitals, we feel desperately, the need to create new training hospitals at new hospitals. There is the known adage that most physicians will end up practicing within 100 miles of where they do their postgraduate training. With the limited number of postgraduate sites—not only in Alaska, but in the Pacific Northwest, that limits the number of recruitment opportunities we have in bringing qualified physicians to Alaska. And, as previously testified, we are always recruiting from outside, we can't produce enough at our current levels to sustain our needs.

Currently, a majority of allopathic and osteopathic residency training programs exist in or near the major metropolitan cities. Dr. Tanner talked about the large number in the State of Texas. And, while those current programs continue to excel at producing high-quality physicians, they don't adequately distribute physicians to communities across the Nation, and particularly to places like Alaska.

A major obstacle often preventing the establishment of new residency training programs, are the costs associated with startup. The AOA proposes the creation of a new program that would assist communities, and rural hospitals, in their efforts to establish new residency training programs.

Under the Physician Workforce and Graduate Medical Education Enhancement Act, the Secretary would be directed to establish an interest-free loan program, whereby hospitals committed to starting a new allopathic or osteopathic residency program, would secure startup funding to offset the initial startup costs. Congress would be asked to allocate adequate money to establish and fund the program. To be eligible, a hospital would demonstrate that they do not currently operate a residency training program, and they must commit to operating a residency program in one of the five medical specialties of primary care—family medicine, internal medicine, pediatrics, OB/GYN, and possibly, general surgery. Hospitals securing a loan under the program would be obliged to repay the total sum, without interest, to the Secretary.

I was just at a meeting last weekend in Portland, the Northwest Osteopathic Conference of States, and there's a small hospital in eastern Oregon who is attempting to start a rural, community-based family practice residency program. And they were there with their CFO, and their hospital administrator, and two of their physicians, basically trying to find out how they were going to come up with the funding to make this work. The desire is there, the need is there. They can't supply their physician staff resources, and they thought with residency training, not only could they grow their own, but they could help offset some of the local physician shortages that already exists. Startup costs are prohibitive. As Dr. Harold Johnston said earlier, our residency program has been operating at a deficit since its inception.

I would say that the Alaska Family Medicine Program has been very kind to us, as an osteopathic professional. They have sought our participation from the beginning, and just last year, hired an osteopathic Physician Director of Medical Education, and that program is now a dually-certified program, so osteopathic medical students can do their residency training at the Family Practice Program and get dual certification from the AOA. And, we are currently, the only operating osteopathic-approved training program in the entire Northwest, at Providence Hospital.

No. 3, Congress should enact legislation that would establish, in statute, clear and concise guidance on the use of ambulatory, non-hospital sites in graduate medical education programs. While the majority of physician training takes place in the hospital setting, it should not be limited to this setting. We need to do more to expose medical students—and resident positions—to different practice settings during their training years. And the Alaska Family Medicine Residency Program has done an excellent job of providing that opportunity.

In 2002, the Centers for Medicare and Medicaid Services began administratively altering the rules. Began denying the time that residents spend in nonhospital settings. As a result, hospitals are being forced to train all residents in the hospital setting, eliminating the valuable, educational experiences offered in the non-hospital training sites. Additionally, some teaching hospitals may be forced to eliminate programs, as a result of the current CMS policies.

Allowing hospitals to receive payments for the time resident physicians train in a nonhospital setting is sound educational policy, and a worthwhile public policy goal that Congress clearly mandated. Additionally, it would be good for us in rural communities.

No. 4, Congress should amend the tax code to allow practicing physicians in rural communities an annual tax credit equal to the amount of interest paid on their student loans. Last year, Senate bill 2789 was introduced, directly addressing tax credits in that regard. I believe you sponsored that legislation. We supported that as an association, and we would support that type of legislation in the future.

We believe this proposal is a direct incentive to young physicians, and would assist in the recruitment and retention of physicians in rural communities.

Additionally, Congress should revise current scholarship, and loan payment programs, to allow physicians to fill their commitment on a part-time basis, as with the National Health Service Corps.

No. 5, Congress should reform the Medicare Physician Payment Formula, by eliminating the sustainable growth rate, and replacing it with a more equitable, and predictable, payment structure. This testimony has already been brought forth. Additionally, Congress should make permanent provisions that establish a floor of 1.0 for their work, geographic practice cost indices, and provide a 5 percent add-on for services provided by physicians, in recognized Medicare-scarcity States, which Alaska certainly is.

Again, we thank you for focusing your attention on this important issue. The AOA, and the AKOMA and our members stand ready to assist you and the committee, as you develop policies aiming at improving access to physicians and physician services. I look forward to your questions.

[The prepared statement of Dr. Perkins follows:]

PREPARED STATEMENT OF BYRON PERKINS, DO

Senator Murkowski and distinguished members of the committee, my name is Byron Perkins. I am a practicing osteopathic family physician in Anchorage and currently serve as the President of the Alaska Osteopathic Medical Association. I am honored to be here today representing the American Osteopathic Association (AOA). The AOA, which represents the Nation's 59,000 osteopathic physicians and over 12,000 osteopathic medical students, applauds the committee's interest in examining this very important issue. Access to physicians and other healthcare services for people residing in rural and other underserved communities is a serious problem. The AOA believes that access to physician services in rural and other underserved communities can be improved by increasing training and workforce opportunities along with developing new programs that aid in the recruitment and placement of osteopathic and allopathic physicians.

We recognize that many communities in the United States face limited access to physicians and physician services. This is especially true in rural and frontier communities. We applaud the efforts made by State governments, the Federal Government, Members of Congress, and rural communities to increase physician access for their citizens. However, like you, we believe much more should be done.

For more than 130 years the AOA and the osteopathic profession has been dedicated to educating and training the future physician workforce. Consistent with our mission, we remain committed to producing primary care physicians who will practice in rural and other underserved communities. This mission has been a tenet of the profession since it's founding in the late 1800's. Today, more than 65 percent of all osteopathic physicians practice in a primary care specialty (family medicine, internal medicine, pediatrics, and obstetrics/gynecology). In Alaska, there are 112 osteopathic physicians. Seventy-two of these osteopathic physicians practice in a primary care specialty, 59 are family physicians [Maps 4 and 5]. Nationwide, more than 100 million patient office visits are made to osteopathic physicians each year.

Over the past 15 years the osteopathic profession has enjoyed tremendous growth. We are one of the fastest growing professions in healthcare. Since 1990 the number of osteopathic physicians has increased 67 percent. Currently, there are 59,000 osteopathic physicians in the United States. The number of osteopathic physicians in the United States is projected to exceed 90,000 by 2015. Osteopathic physicians represent 6 percent of the current U.S. physician workforce and over 8 percent of all military physicians.

Throughout our history, the osteopathic profession has placed an emphasis on primary care and rural service. Our commitment to these goals is reflected in our membership and in the mission statements of the Nation's colleges of osteopathic medicine. Our emphasis on primary care and rural practice is reflected by the fact that currently 22 percent of osteopathic physicians practice in a designated medically underserved area (MUA) (Map 1). As our membership grows, the AOA is refocusing its efforts on our core mission—training physicians who are capable and willing to provide high quality care to our Nation's neediest populations.

The issues facing our Nation's rural healthcare system are complex. We do not suggest that there are easy answers, but we do believe that change in some policies would increase our ability to meet these needs.

The following pages outline several recommendations. These recommendations would improve the ability of the AOA and our allopathic colleagues to meet the needs of rural and other underserved communities. We believe that the implementation of these recommendations will allow the U.S. medical education system to meet its responsibilities of training physicians who will provide quality healthcare to all populations regardless of their geographic location.

PHYSICIAN WORKFORCE

Many experts now believe that the United States will face a shortfall in its physician supply over the next 20 years. While academic and policy experts debate the needs and expectations of the future physician workforce, the AOA recognizes that we must begin to educate and train a larger cadre of physicians, now.

The time it takes to educate and train a physician is, at minimum, 7 years. This means that a student accepted in the matriculating class of 2007 will not enter the physician workforce until at least 2014. Due to the time required to educate and train future physicians, we believe a concentrated effort must be focused on increasing the Nation's physician education and post-graduate training capacity over the next 5 years. If handled appropriately, the country could increase the physician workforce dramatically by 2020.

Reliance upon the J-1 Visa program is neither the most effective nor the most desirable way to increase physician supply in rural communities, although we recognize that the program can provide short-term relief. The J-1 program is not capable of meeting the physician workforce needs of our Nation and should not be promoted for this purpose. Yes, a few States and communities have physician services as a result of the J-1 program. However, thousands of rural communities remain without physician services. The AOA supports increasing our capacity by adopting policies that encourage larger numbers of U.S.-educated and trained physicians to practice in rural and underserved areas. An increase in U.S.-educated and trained physicians, if properly selected and trained, will lead to a more predictable and reliable physician workforce and is more likely to produce larger numbers of physicians who will practice in rural communities.

Today, one in five medical students in the United States is enrolled in a college of osteopathic medicine. Fifty percent of the students enrolled in the Nation's colleges of osteopathic medicine are women. Currently, there are 23 colleges of osteopathic medicine operating on 26 campuses (See Map 2). There are two additional colleges that will open within the next 2 years, bringing the total number of colleges to 25 that are operating on 28 campuses. In 2007, these colleges will graduate approximately 3,000 new osteopathic physicians. In 2008, the number of graduates will increase to 3,500. By 2013 the number of osteopathic physicians graduating from colleges of osteopathic medicine is projected to reach 4,500. Assuming a predictable growth pattern, the osteopathic profession should produce approximately 5,000 new physicians per year beginning in 2015.

The current colleges of osteopathic medicine, and those set to open in the future, are located in regions that historically have had limited access to physician services. Currently, there are three colleges of osteopathic medicine in Appalachian region, one in Las Vegas and one developing in Denver—two of the Nation's fastest growing communities, three colleges in the States of Missouri and Oklahoma, and Yakima, Washington—which aims to meet the needs of several Northwest States including Alaska. The location of current and future colleges of osteopathic medicine reflects the osteopathic profession's commitment to rural and underserved communities.

In Alaska, we are especially proud of the Pacific Northwest University of Health Sciences (PNUHS) in Yakima, Washington, which will begin classes in 2008. Along with my colleagues in Alaska, I am optimistic that PNUHS will begin contributing to Alaska's physician workforce in the near future. The AOA urges the Alaska legislature to develop new programs that encourage a significant number of Alaska residents to pursue their medical education at the PNUHS College of Osteopathic Medicine.

INTERNATIONAL MEDICAL GRADUATES

The U.S. healthcare system is widely recognized as the most advanced in the world. The rapid development of new diagnoses and treatments outpaces those in other countries. We are the world's leader in medicine and medical technology. In this role, we should share our expertise with the world. For this reason, the AOA supports the continued acceptance of international medical graduates (IMGs) into the U.S.-graduate medical education system. By training international physicians, we can improve the healthcare delivery systems around the world by improving the quality of the physicians. However, this transfer of knowledge and skills cannot take place if international physicians do not return to their home countries.

The United States should not be an importer of physicians. The majority of international physicians should come to the United States to train and then return home. The "brain drain" in many countries is well documented. Many countries lose their best and brightest young physicians to the United States and other English-speaking countries. International physicians should come here to train and should not be encouraged to stay upon completion of their training. In fact, we should require that they return to their home countries and practice medicine for an extended period of time before they are eligible to petition for a visa, J-1 or otherwise.

In 2006, almost 9,000 IMGs participated in the National Residency Matching Program (NRMP). Of these applicants, approximately 6,500 were not U.S. citizens and 2,500 were U.S. citizens who attended a foreign medical school. Almost 50 percent of all IMGs match to first year residency positions. In 2006, the total number of IMGs who matched to first year positions increased to 4,382.

Of the 6,500 IMG participants who were not U.S. citizens, 3,151 (48.9 percent) obtained first year positions. 2006 was the fifth consecutive year that the number of non-U.S. citizen IMGs matching to first year positions increased. Of the 2,500 U.S. citizen IMG participants, 1,231 (50.6 percent) were matched to first year positions. 2006 was the third consecutive year that the number of U.S. citizen IMGs matching to first year positions increased. The total number of IMGs filling first year residency positions will be much higher than the approximate 4,400 who secured positions through the NRMP. Many IMGs are able to secure residency training positions outside the match.

RECRUITMENT AND PLACEMENT

Medical schools and colleges of osteopathic medicine traditionally place significant emphasis on an applicant's academic achievement—grade point average, undergraduate degree program, and scores on the Medical College Admission Test (MCAT). While we would never suggest that the academic standards required for admittance be lowered, we do recommend that the Nation's medical education institutions begin evaluating "other" factors. An evaluation of the student's life, including an evaluation of where the student was raised, attended high school, and location of family members, provides an indication of where a future physician may practice. For example, an applicant from Manhattan, New York is less likely to practice in a rural community than an applicant from Manhattan, Kansas. If the two applicants are equally qualified, we should encourage our schools to matriculate the student from Manhattan, Kansas, an individual more likely to return to rural Kansas once education and training is completed.

Our medical education system must increase its efforts to promote both primary care specialties and experience in rural practice locations. Over the years, the role of the rural family physician became less glamorous than that of the urban subspecialist. Far too many medical school students want to be an "ologist" instead of a general surgeon, family physician, general internist, or pediatrician. Our Nation's healthcare system needs specialists and subspecialists, but we need far more primary care physicians. Our medical education system must place greater emphasis on educating and training primary care physicians and general surgeons. These physicians are more likely to practice in a rural or small community hospital and are far more likely to practice in rural America.

The AOA believes that programs funded and operated under Title VII of the Public Health Service Act are essential to achieving the goals outlined above. Over the past 5 years, title VII programs have seen a dramatic decrease in both support and funding. We urge Congress to reverse this trend and place greater emphasis on these important programs.

INCREASE TRAINING CAPACITY

Currently, there are approximately 96,000 funded residency positions in the United States. The number of funded residency positions has been static since the late 1990's when Congress, as part of the Balanced Budget Act of 1997, placed a limit or "caps" on the number of funded residency slots any existing teaching program may have.

The residency caps were established at a time when the general consensus was that the country had an adequate supply of physicians. We now recognize this is not correct. The residency caps established by the BBA limit the ability of teaching hospitals to increase training programs, thus preventing responsible growth capable of meeting our future physician workforce needs. The AOA encourages Congress to either remove or increase the caps on the number of funded graduate medical education training "slots" as established by the Balanced Budget Act of 1997.

This past week, Senators Harry Reid and Bill Nelson introduced the "Resident Physician Shortage Reduction Act of 2007." This legislation authorizes the Secretary of the Department of Health and Human Services (HHS) to increase the number of residency cap positions for which Medicare payments will be made if certain criteria are met. The increases or cap adjustments target teaching hospitals in eligible States where there is a demonstrated shortage of resident physicians. States would be considered to have a shortage of resident physicians if its ratio of allopathic and osteopathic physicians training in ACGME or AOA approved residency and/or fellowship programs is below the national median number per 100,000 population. According to current statistics, the national median number of resident physicians per 100,000 population is 25. Teaching hospitals in 24 States would be allowed to increase their FTE cap under the proposed formula.

The AOA supports this legislation and urges all Senators to cosponsor this important bill. Furthermore, we call upon the Senate to approve this legislation this year.

IMPROVE RURAL TRAINING PROGRAMS

There is an old saying in medical education circles that physicians will practice within 100 miles of where they train. While the validity of this saying either in a world that is limited to the United States' borders or alternatively in an era of globalization is unproven, its message rings true. Physicians are more likely to practice in settings where they have the most experience. While a majority of physician training takes place in the hospital setting, it should not be limited to this setting. We need to do more to expose medical students and resident physicians to different practice settings during their training years.

A valuable component of graduate medical education is the experience of training at nonhospital ambulatory sites. These sites include physician offices, nursing homes, and community health centers. Ambulatory training sites provide an important educational experience because of the broad range of patients and conditions treated and by ensuring that residents are exposed to practice settings similar to those in which they ultimately may practice. This type of training is particularly important for primary care residency programs since a majority of these physicians will practice in nonhospital ambulatory clinics upon completion of their training. This training also is essential to improving access to care in rural communities.

Congress has long recognized that a greater focus should be placed on training physicians in rural and other underserved communities. In the 1990s, Congress began to fear that the current graduate medical education payment formula discouraged the training of resident physicians in ambulatory settings. This opinion was based upon the fact that the payment formula only accounted for the resident training time in a hospital setting.

Through the Balanced Budget Act of 1997, Congress altered the payment formula, removing the disincentives that existed for training in nonhospital settings. We accomplished this goal by allowing hospitals to count the training time of residents in nonhospital settings for the purpose of including such time in their Medicare cost reports for both indirect medical education (IME) and direct graduate medical education (DGME) payments.

This change in the payment formula was designed to increase the amount of training a resident physician received in nonhospital settings, enhance access to care for patients in rural and other underserved communities, provide an additional education experience for residents who are considering practicing in rural communities, and provide a recruitment mechanism for rural and underserved communities in need of physicians.

The program appeared to be working as intended. However, in 2002 the Centers for Medicare and Medicaid Services (CMS) began administratively altering the rules and regulations in respect to this issue. As a result, CMS intermediaries began denying the time residents spent in nonhospital settings. In many cases, hospitals were forced to repay thousands of dollars as a result of this administrative change in regulations.

Many Members of Congress urged CMS to work with interested parties to resolve this issue by developing new regulations that clarify the appropriate use of nonhospital settings. Unfortunately, these conversations have not produced policies that meet the original intent of Congress as established in 1997. As a result, hospitals are being forced to train all residents in the hospital setting, eliminating the valuable educational experiences offered in nonhospital training sites. Additionally, some teaching hospitals may be forced to eliminate residency programs entirely as a result of current CMS policies.

Allowing hospitals to receive payments for the time resident physicians train in a nonhospital setting is sound educational policy and a worthwhile public policy goal that Congress clearly mandated in 1997. Additionally, it is good for rural communities.

DEVELOPMENT OF NEW TEACHING HOSPITALS

In addition to expanding the training capacity at existing teaching hospitals, we desperately need to create new training programs at new hospitals. Currently, a majority of allopathic and osteopathic residency training programs exist in or near the major metropolitan cities on the east coast, west coast, and Great Lakes region. While the current programs continue to excel at producing high quality physicians, they do not adequately distribute physicians to communities across the Nation.

As we outlined previously, it is well documented that physicians establish practices near the location of their training program. Assuming this to be true, the Nation desperately needs new training programs in many States, especially those in the Midwest, Southwest, Northwest, and Rocky Mountain regions. By providing greater number of residency training programs in these areas, the physician workforce shortage could be reduced greatly for many States.

A major obstacle often preventing the establishment of new residency training programs are the costs associated with the creation of such programs. Under current law, a hospital starting a new residency program is not eligible for direct graduate medical education (DGME) or indirection medical education (IME) funding until they have filed their initial cost-report with the Centers for Medicare and Medicaid Services (CMS). Initial cost reports are filed following the completion of the first year the residency program is in operation. The first payments from CMS to hospitals with new residency programs typically occurs around 16 to 18 months after the program is started. This financing arrangement presents challenges for hospitals that operate on narrow margins, especially community hospitals that lack adequate reserve funds to offset the financial commitments associated with starting a new residency program.

The AOA is working with Members of Congress to develop a new program that would assist community and rural hospitals in their efforts to establish new residency training programs. Under the "Physician Workforce and Graduate Medical Education Enhancement Act," the Secretary would be directed to establish an interest-free loan program whereby hospitals committed to starting new osteopathic or allopathic residency training programs could secure startup funding to offset the initial costs of starting such programs. Congress would be asked to allocate adequate money to establish and fund the program.

To be eligible, a hospital must demonstrate that they currently do not operate a residency training program, have not operated a residency training program in the past, and that they have secured preliminary accreditation by the American Council on Graduate Medical Education (ACGME) and/or the American Osteopathic Association (AOA). Additionally, the petitioning hospital must commit to operating an allopathic or osteopathic residency program in one of five medical specialties or a combination of these specialties: family medicine, internal medicine, emergency medicine, obstetrics/gynecology, or general surgery.

A hospital may request funding to assist in the development of a residency training program. We suggest that the financing be limited to no more than $1 million. Funding could be used to offset the costs of residency salaries and benefits, faculty salaries, and other costs directly attributable to the residency program.

Hospitals securing a loan under the program would be obligated to repay the total sum, without interest, to the Secretary. Hospitals would have two repayment options—repayment in full or repayment through a financing mechanism. The AOA looks forward to working with Members of the U.S. Senate on this concept and is optimistic that this type of a program would enhance the disbursement of physicians to communities in need.

EXPAND PROGRAMS THAT PROVIDE INCENTIVES FOR RURAL PRACTICE

There are numerous existing programs that provide scholarships and loan repayment for physicians who choose to practice in rural communities. These programs include the National Health Service Corps, Public Health Service, Indian Health Service, and many programs operated by State governments. The AOA supports these programs and encourages Congress to continue funding them at levels that facilitate greater numbers of physicians practicing in rural and other underserved communities.

Additionally, we believe that some consideration should be given to allow physicians to participate in the programs on a part-time basis. There are numerous communities that need physician services, but they may not need them full time. We believe that modifications should be made to Federal loan repayment and scholarship programs that allow participants to repay on a part-time basis in exchange for a longer term of service. For example, if a physician participates in the National Health Service Corps and agrees to a 3-year commitment in a rural community— why not allow the physician the option of committing to 4 or 5 year's service on a part-time basis. We believe this would encourage more physicians to participate in these valuable programs without jeopardizing the underlying mission.

The AOA also proposes a change in the tax code that would provide physicians practicing in designated rural communities with a tax credit equal to the amount of interest paid on their student loans for any given year that they practice in such a community, or until their loans are paid in full. Under current law, individuals may deduct up to $2,500 in interest paid on student loans from their Federal income taxes. However, the income thresholds associated with this provision often prevent physicians from qualifying. Our proposal would provide a direct link between practice location and the tax credit. A physician practicing in rural Wyoming who pays $8,000 in interest on her student loans in year one would get an $8,000 tax credit for that year. The program would continue until the physicians had retired her student loan debt or when she departed the rural community. We believe that this proposal provides a direct incentive to young physicians and would assist in the recruitment and retention of physicians in rural communities.

IMPROVE THE ECONOMICS OF MEDICINE

The current practice environment physicians face is challenging. Over the past decade escalating professional liability insurance premiums, decreasing reimbursements, and expanded regulations have made the practice of medicine more frustrating for all physicians. These issues are compounded in rural communities where physicians are often in solo practice or small group practices, unable to benefit from economies of scale that larger group practices in urban areas enjoy.

According to a 2004 Health Affairs study, more than half of all practicing physicians are in practices of three or fewer physicians. Three-quarters are in practices of eight or fewer. They face the same economic barriers as every other small business in America. Costs associated with staff salaries; health and other benefits, basic medical supplies, and technology, all essential components of any business, continue to rise at a rate that far outpaces reimbursements. When facing deep reductions in reimbursements at the same time that their operational costs are increasing, it is safe to project that most businesses will not be able to continue operation. While most businesses increase, or have the ability to increase, their prices to make up the differential between costs and reimbursements, physicians participating in Medicare cannot.

- *Physician Payment*—Since 2001, Medicare physician payment rates have fallen greater than 20 percent below the Government's measure of inflation in medical practice costs. In 2002, physicians' payments under Medicare were cut 5.4 percent.
- If the projected cuts are implemented, the average physician payment rate will be less in 2007 than it was in 2001. Additionally, two provisions included in the Medicare Modernization Act (MMA), which provide increased reimbursements for physicians in rural communities, will expire over the next 2 years.
- In 2002, physician payments were cut by 5.4 percent. Congress acted to avert payment cuts in 2003, 2004, 2005, 2006, and 2007 replacing projected cuts of approximately 5 percent per year with increases of 1.6 percent in 2003, 1.5 percent in 2004 and 2005, and 0 percent in 2006 and 2007. Even with these increases, physician payments fell further behind medical practice costs. Practice costs from 2002 through 2006 were about two times the amount of payment increases. The long-term projections are even more startling. Under the current formula, physicians face cuts of greater than 30 percent over the next 8 years.
- Since its inception in 1965, a central tenet of the Medicare program is the physician-patient relationship. Medicare beneficiaries rely upon physicians for access to

all other aspects of the Medicare program. This relationship has become compromised by dramatic reductions in reimbursements, increased regulatory burdens, and escalating practice costs. These projected cuts come at a time when the number of Medicare beneficiaries is projected to grow from the current 43 million to more than 71 million. Additionally, since many healthcare programs, such as TRICARE, Medicaid, and private insurers link their payments to Medicare rates, cuts in other systems will compound the impact of the projected Medicare cuts. Medicare cuts actually trigger cuts in other programs.

• Additional cuts in Medicare physician payments threaten Medicare beneficiaries' ability to access to physician services. These access problems are compounded in rural communities where the loss of a single physician can equate to no access for beneficiaries in that community. These problems will only increase if additional cuts are implemented.

• Furthermore, reduced payments hamper the ability of physicians to purchase and implement new technologies in their practices. According to a 2005 study published in *Health Affairs*, the average costs of implementing electronic health records was $44,000 per full-time equivalent provider, with ongoing costs of $8,500 per provider per year for maintenance of the system. This is not an insignificant investment. When facing deep reductions in reimbursements, it is safe to project that physicians will be prohibited financially from adopting and implementing new technologies.

• Physician payments should reflect increases in practice costs. Now is the time to establish a stable, predictable, and accurate physician payment formula that reflects the cost of providing care.

• Congress must act to reform the Medicare physician payment formula. Continued use of the flawed SGR formula will have a negative impact upon patient access to care. Additionally, Congress should act to extend expiring provisions that provide incentives to physicians in rural communities. The Medicare Modernization Act (MMA) altered the Medicare physician payment formula by establishing a 1.0 floor for the work geographic practice cost indices (GPCI) under the Medicare physician fee schedule and created a 5 percent add-on payment for physicians practicing in recognized Medicare physician scarcity areas. The MMA reversed years of inequities in payments between rural physicians and those in larger urban communities. Congress extended the 1.0 floor for the work GPCI as part of the "Tax Relief and Health Care Act of 2006" (H.R. 6111). However, both the GPCI and Medicare scarcity provisions expire on December 31, 2007 unless Congress acts. We believe that these are essential and positive Medicare payment policies that should be extended, if not made permanent. Both provisions will enhance beneficiary access and improve the quality of care available.

• *Medical Liability Reform*—As you know, the Nation's medical liability system is broken. In recent years physicians across the Nation have faced escalating professional liability insurance premiums. According to the National Association of Insurance Commissioners (NAIC), between 1975 and 2002 medical liability premiums for physicians increased, on average, 750 percent. These premium increases are related directly to an explosion in medical liability lawsuits filed against physicians and hospitals and the rapid increase in awards. The Government Accountability Office (GAO) confirms this. In a 2003 report, the GAO stated that losses on medical liability claims are the primary driver of increases in medical liability insurance premiums.

• As a result of a broken medical liability system patients face reduced access to healthcare, the overall costs of healthcare increases, and the future supply of physicians is threatened. Many physicians no longer provide services that are deemed high-risk, such as delivering babies, covering emergency departments, or performing certain surgical procedures. This crisis also impacts primary care physicians, especially those in rural areas who are often the only physician practicing in a community. As a result, patients have seen a decrease in the availability of physician services. Additionally, the medical liability crisis has a significant impact upon the career choices of future physicians. In a recent poll conducted by the AOA, 82 percent of osteopathic medical students stated that the cost and availability of medical liability insurance would influence their future specialty choices, while 86 percent stated that it would influence their decision on where to establish a practice once their training was complete. This trend in career choices is disturbing and will have a long-term impact upon the healthcare delivery system in the years ahead.

SUMMARY

Again, the AOA appreciates the opportunity to share our views on this important issue. We remain committed to working with Congress to enact legislation that will ensure access to quality physician services for all Americans, regardless of where they reside. In closing we would like to highlight five recommendations made in our testimony that we believe will lead to improved access to physician services, increase the availability of U.S.-trained physicians, improve the quality of training for future physicians, and improve the recruitment and retention of physicians in rural communities.

1. Congress should consider eliminating the cap on available and funded residency positions in the United States. This cap hinders the ability of osteopathic and allopathic medical schools to educate and train larger numbers of physicians. To meet the healthcare needs of our growing population we must have the capacity and financing to train a larger number of physicians. The AOA supports the "Resident Physician Shortage Reduction Act of 2007" and urges the Senate to approve this legislation in 2007.

2. Congress should establish and fund a new interest-free loan program to assist in the creation of new residency training programs at hospitals that have not operated teaching programs previously. By expanding opportunities to new hospitals, Congress can facilitate the training of physicians in new geographic regions that currently have limited access to physicians.

3. Congress should enact legislation that would establish, in statute, clear and concise guidance on the use of ambulatory nonhospital sites in graduate medical education programs. If enacted, it will preserve the quality education of resident physicians originally envisioned by Congress in 1997.

4. Congress should amend the tax code to allow physicians practicing in rural communities an annual tax credit equal to the amount of interest paid on their student loans. We believe that this proposal provides a direct incentive to young physicians and would assist in the recruitment and retention of physicians in rural communities. Additionally, Congress should revise current scholarship and loan repayment programs to allow physicians to fulfill their commitment on a part-time basis.

5. Congress should reform the Medicare physician payment formula by eliminating the sustainable growth rate and replacing it with a more equitable and predictable payment structure. Additionally, Congress should make permanent provisions that establish a floor of 1.0 for the work of GPCI and provide a 5 percent add-on for services provided by physicians in recognized Medicare scarcity areas.

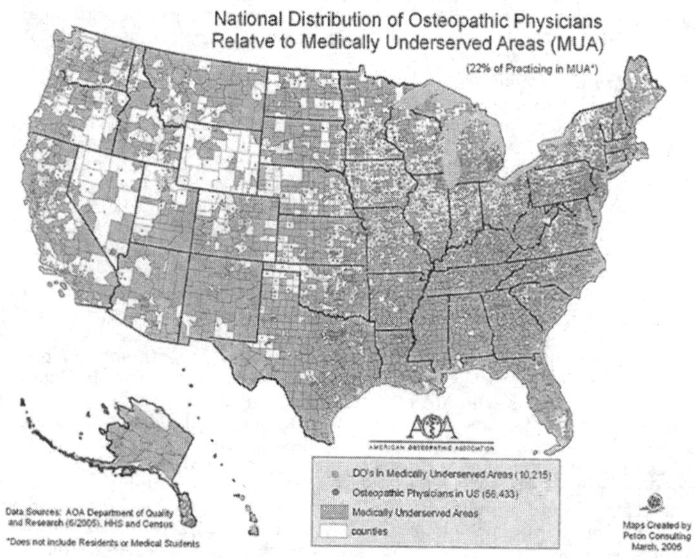

[Map 1] National Distribution of Osteopathic Physicians Relative to Medically Underserved Areas

Colleges of Osteopathic Medicine

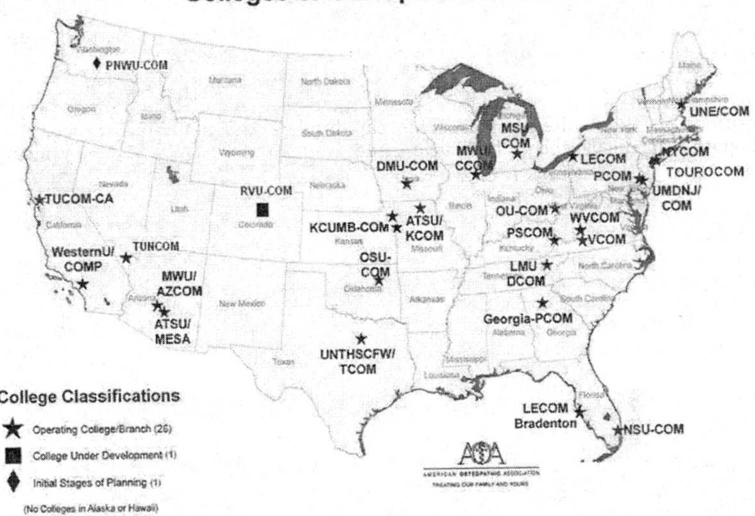

[Map 2] Colleges of Osteopathic Medicine

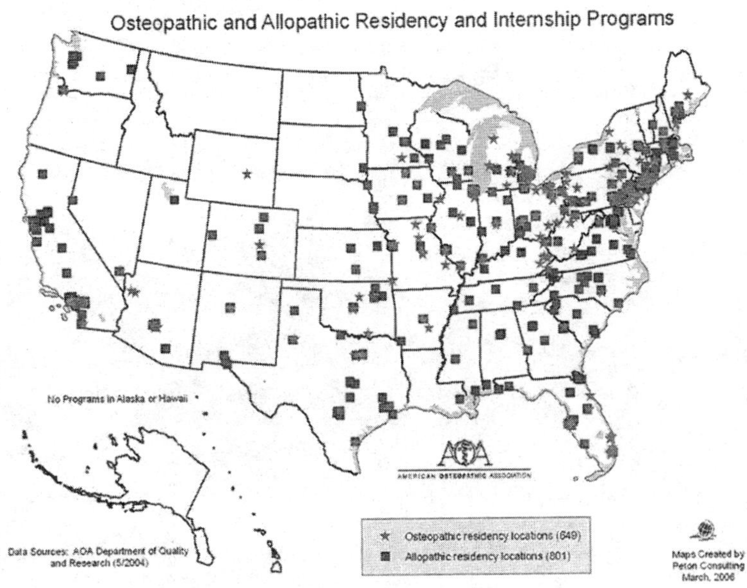

[Map 3] Osteopathic and Allopathic Residency and Internship Programs

112 Alaska Osteopathic Physicians

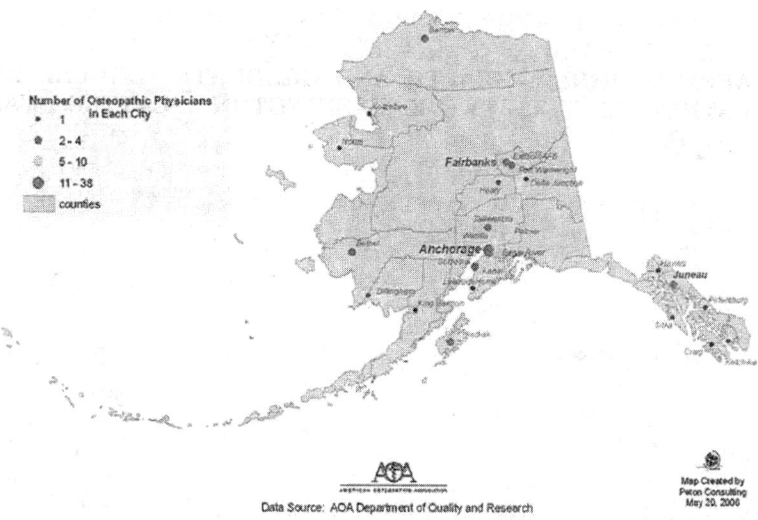

[Map 4] Osteopathic Physicians in Alaska

72 Primary Care Osteopathic Physicians in Alaska

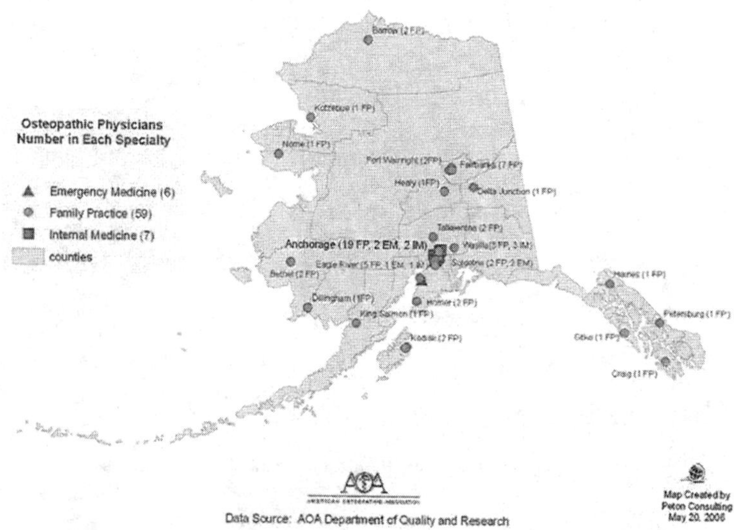

[Map 5] Primary Care Osteopathic Physicians in Alaska

Senator MURKOWSKI. Thank you, Doctor.

Next, let's go to Dr. Coombs, University of Washington School of Medicine. Tell us a little bit about WWAMI this morning.

STATEMENT OF JOHN COOMBS, ASSOCIATE VICE-PRESIDENT FOR MEDICAL AFFAIRS, ASSOCIATE DEAN FOR REGIONAL AFFAIRS, RURAL HEALTH AND GRADUATE MEDICAL EDUCATION, UNIVERSITY OF WASHINGTON, SEATTLE, WASHINGTON

Dr. COOMBS. Thank you, Senator Murkowski. And I want to also express my appreciation on the part of the HELP Committee—Health, Education, Labor, and Pensions—for inviting testimony today from the WWAMI program. I want to try to summarize some of my written comments that I have brought forward, in the interest of also having questions that you might bring forward, and to address beyond what we have said today.

What is really remarkable to me is that when I began at the WWAMI Program at its inception, actually, 35 years ago, I was a practicing rural family physician in a very small community in north-central Washington, a National Health Service Corps volunteer, and someone who now has built upon that experience to continue to pledge our efforts, in terms of the University of Washington School of Medicine and WWAMI, into meeting future needs for physicians practicing in those areas.

In your opening comments, you mentioned that the size of the rural population in the United States is roughly about 21 percent of our total population. In the WWAMI area, that number, actually, is 35 percent, and in Alaska, it's greater than 50 percent of the population of the State of Alaska, who live in rural communities, and in Wyoming, Montana and Idaho, the number is even greater than 50 percent. So, this is a significant issue, in terms of the WWAMI Program.

The thing I want to emphasize today, is the success of the WWAMI Program has been, really, predicated by partnership. The partnership that has existed between the Alaska State legislature, and the other legislatures across the five States among the institutions of higher education, such as the University of Alaska, Anchorage. Also, among practicing physicians, such as the Alaska State Medical Association and the volunteerism that goes forward to teach our students and residents. Also, among the hospitals within the State, who have put forward resource and energy to allow for the training of future physicians within those areas, as well as direct support for programs such as residency training. And also, among the partnership that exists between WWAMI and the Federal Government. And that really is the issue that I'd like to specifically center on today.

Over the course of the past decade, the number of physicians entering family medicine from the WWAMI Program has gone from 36 percent of the graduating class, to this year, an anticipated 12 percent. Similarly, during that time, primary care has dropped from over 60 percent, to now just greater than 38 percent. As a consequence, as you can see, the shortage that we're facing, we're not directing physicians in the way that we intend to, which is toward careers in primary healthcare.

And why is this? Many of these issues have been mentioned today, but the mounting student debt, the shortage of really a critical unit in terms of being able to have adequate physicians within isolated communities, as well as large, urban communities. In addition to the absence of adequate applicants to residency programs who have done their training in the United States, which now, across the Nation, is less than 49 percent of U.S. medical school graduates now fill our Family Practice Residency Programs, as an example.

This is a significant issue. What can we do about this, in terms of the restoration of this in terms of the Federal partnership that we have within WWAMI? First of all, we need to restore and enlarge support for student debt relief. I think the National Health Service Corps—and particularly, I was pleased in your opening comments to hear you say, "the relationship between academic training programs, and community health centers"—there needs to be a stronger community/academic partnership which is developed that will allow for the training of family physicians, primary care internists, general pediatricians, general surgeons, and psychiatrists within settings such as that, to meet future needs, and access to care for people in isolated areas.

The second thing is, that we need to fix the overall healthcare delivery system to create greater incentive for primary care physicians, and this has been mentioned by my colleagues who have testified before.

At the present time, the financial incentive, or disincentive, to enter into primary care is very remarkable, in terms of the onus that this places upon medical students who are now facing, on our situation, $94,000 debt from people who graduate from the WWAMI Program who are from Alaska, in comparison to $125,000 that was mentioned earlier from public medical schools, and between $150,000 and $200,000 from private medical schools.

We need to maintain and to incent training for primary care, and the essential specialties. And to do this, I want to make 8 points from the Federal perspective, that would help.

First, is to eliminate caps for these primary care specialties in areas such as the critical things such as general surgery, and psychiatry. To enable hospitals and people who support graduate medical education, to build additional capacity in that respect.

Second, not to allow for further reduction, and to restore reductions in Medicare and Medicaid that support graduate medical education, and medical education in general. This also includes the appropriated funds for pediatric training, and graduate medical education, which are currently scheduled for substantial reduction in this year's considerations.

We need to increase the training for opportunities for residents in the critical needs specialties, and to build upon things—even in States like Alaska that do not, perhaps, have their own programs— we need to be innovative in terms of placing general surgeons, psychiatrists and internists, such as we have done in the State of Idaho, for instance, through the WWAMI Program, to bring them to Alaska as well, and to create innovative programs that will allow us to do that.

We need to restore title VII funding. Currently that is pegged with the budgetary considerations to basically be eliminated this year. And this is something which supports our residency training, our medical student training, our faculty development, and a number of other areas which are essential, as far as the success that WWAMI has created over the course of the past 35 years.

We need to restore the Health Careers Opportunities Program, HCOP, so that we can take people who come from underserved communities such as many of the areas in Alaska, to bring them to medical school, and to bring them into the health professions. Currently, in Dr. Johnston's program, there are two people who have participated in the HCOP Program within WWAMI who are now residents here. But, that program now has been eliminated. And so, what are we going to do to reach out to Alaska's communities, to bring people to healthcare careers in the future, and to just tell them, simply, "You can do it." And we're here to help them make that happen.

We need to expand funding for the National Health Service Corps Scholarship Program, which has been very effective. Dr. Johnston was also a National Health Service Corps volunteer, and someone who was brought into medicine through that mechanism. We need to restore funding for the Bureau of Health Professions, for the Center for Health Workforce Studies across the country, such that we can evaluate innovative programs and estimate the needs. That has now been eliminated over the course of the past 2 years, through the Bureau of Healthcare Professions.

And, finally, I want to come back to creating this academic community health center alliance, where we can begin to have training programs within these CHCs, to be able to bring trainees to them, and to actually create the success that I think can be done in that respect.

This is a long list of things, in terms of the Federal support. But, it is something that I want to return to the fact that, partnership has been the thing that has led to the success of WWAMI.

I've provided in my written testimony, information which is available to you, and other members of the HELP Committee, including our continuum of medical education, which really brings out all of the programs which rely upon Federal support in terms of their continuance. Much of which, now, has been eliminated.

Finally, now, I just want to briefly touch upon the success that WWAMI has created. The Program has been successful, not only because of this partnership, but it's bringing incredibly capable students from States such as Alaska into the opportunity to achieve publicly-supported medical education. We're joined today, if they could stand, by the students who are currently in the pipeline of WWAMI from Alaska, who are going to be the future of healthcare delivery in Alaska.

[Applause.]

For every student who just stood, there are six other qualified students who could be here today, if there was just the resources to be able to bring them into the pipeline. And also, to be able to enlarge upon the graduate medical education programs that exist within the State.

The student return rate for WWAMI is 61 percent who return to WWAMI to practice medicine. This is a remarkable thing, especially when you look at the State of Alaska, where 47 percent of those who start in the State of Alaska return, but 84 percent of the positions, the 10 positions per year, are filled by students who have graduated from WWAMI, who return to the State to practice.

The second thing is that WWAMI is very cost-effective. Our tuition, the $15,900 per year, is $4,000 below the National average for public medical schools. And so, not only is that something that is cost-effective, but also, the total cost of educating students of—what seems like an enormous amount of money—of $57,000, is far below the average of $60,000 to $120,000 nationally, to educate medical students.

We've been fortunate to be named the number one primary care medical school in the United States by *U.S. News & World Report*, for the last 13 years. No. 1 in family medicine, number one in rural health. But, I think the critical issue is, we need to have the support of all of the partners to be able to continue to do this.

We've been fortunate that through the program, such as Dr. Johnston's Family Practice Residency Program, 77 percent of the 350 residents who are part of that Program, have returned to practice in WWAMI. And, among those, 30 percent in communities of less than 25,000, 15 percent in communities of less than 5,000. So, we need to continue to be able to innovate.

So, I'd like to just conclude by saying, again, thank you very much to the HELP Committee for allowing me to come and testify, and share with you some of the success of WWAMI, but also, to encourage us to return to the partnership that has made us successful, and has benefited the people of, not only the State of Alaska, but across the WWAMI region, and the Nation, in terms of the preparation of future family physicians, and physicians in other specialties.

Thank you.

[The prepared statement of Dr. Coombs follows:]

PREPARED STATEMENT OF JOHN B. COOMBS, M.D.

My name is John Coombs and I am a physician on the faculty at the University of Washington School of Medicine. As a family physician and pediatrician and as a member of the Dean's office, my responsibilities include the oversight of the WWAMI Program.

Today it is my privilege to testify before you from my leadership position in the WWAMI Program. As I will outline below, WWAMI (Washington, Wyoming, Alaska, Montana, Idaho) has accomplished much in its nearly 35 years of serving the region. From a Federal perspective, I can say that we have only been able to accomplish this record with continuing Federal support. We have partnered with the Federal Government all along the way and I want to begin by thanking this committee and the programs it funds for the support you have given to WWAMI over the years.

At the end of my testimony, I will suggest specific ways that we together can reinvigorate our partnership. Recent years have seen a decline in Federal support for what we do. While we appreciate the realities of the Federal budget, I hope to convince you that your investments in support of medical education are key to managing the physician crisis in rural America, the subject of this hearing.

WWAMI stands for Washington, Wyoming, Alaska, Montana and Idaho. The University of Washington School of Medicine is the only medical school and academic medical center within this five-State area. The region comprises approximately 27 percent of the total land mass of the United States. The approximately 10 million people in the region constitute 3 percent of the population in the United States. Thirty-five percent of the people living within this five-State region live in rural communities. This year we are celebrating the 35th anniversary of WWAMI, and are acknowledging the remarkable interstate partnership that has been developed to allow for public access to medical school for the citizens of the five States. This has only been possible through the cooperative relationship between the people of the five States and the medical school. This is a relationship which has evolved between institutions of higher education, physicians in practice, hospitals, and the State legislatures as we work together to support, in an enduring fashion, this remarkable partnership.

In each of the past 14 years, the University of Washington School of Medicine and the WWAMI Program have been recognized by *U.S. News & World Report* as the No. 1 Medical School in the United States in primary care as well as in rural health and Family Medicine. Though the program began with a focus solely on training medical students, our evolution has been toward the development of a continuum of educational services (represented in the attachments as the "WWAMI Educational Continuum") that begins before medical school and extends into community service. It has also evolved into the creation of graduate medical education programs that have allowed for graduates of WWAMI to continue on with their training within the five-State area in family medicine, pediatrics, internal Medicine and psychiatry. In 2002, the Association of American Medical Colleges recognized WWAMI with its prestigious Outstanding Community Service Award, applauding the partnership between the UWSOM and communities within WWAMI.

The material that I have provided to you as part of this testimony is the current Executive Summary of Activities in the States of Alaska and Wyoming over the past 12 months. The insert to both of these reports provides a State map, which allows for visual representation of communities where the WWAMI program is based within the States. In addition, on the back of the map page is a pictorial representation of the WWAMI Educational Continuum. This material will give the reader an in-depth glimpse of exactly what WWAMI does within the States of Alaska and Wyoming.

Overall, the outcomes of the program are substantial. Sixty-one percent of our medical students have returned to practice within the five-State WWAMI area. This compares favorably to the national average return rate (for all medical schools) return rate of 41 percent. In addition, over the course of the past 20 years, approximately 40 percent–55 percent of graduates have entered into residencies in primary care (national average, 7 percent–10 percent). Over a similar timeframe, 15 percent–30 percent of WWAMI graduates have chosen to establish practices in rural and medically underserved areas. Hence, WWAMI ranks highly among the States with regards to return of graduates to practice within the communities where they trained. Similarly, WWAMI ranks highly in providing well-trained physicians ready for primary care careers in rural and medically underserved communities. The Family Practice Residency Network, which is affiliated with the University of Washington and brings together 17 Family Practice Programs across the five States (one of which is here in Anchorage), has a return rate of 77 percent of graduates to practice within the five-State area. Of these graduates, 30 percent practice in communities of less than 25,000 and 15 percent in communities of less than 5,000 people—most often in communities that are medically underserved and/or rural. Additional information is provided on the State-specific Fact Sheets that are attached to this testimony in conjunction with the Executive Summary Reports.

The WWAMI Program is remarkably cost-effective. The total cost to States averages between $45,000–$55,000 per student, per year for medical student education within WWAMI. This compares favorably to national averages of $60,000 and $120,000 per student, per year in medical schools in States outside of the WWAMI region. In addition, the tuition that is paid by students at the University of Washington School of Medicine is $15,900 per year, approximately $4,000 less than the national average among publicly supported medical schools. This cost effectiveness is consistent with one of the original 1970 goals of the WWAMI Program which was to assist WWAMI States in avoiding duplicative capital costs and the expenses of hiring new faculty. The WWAMI Program would not have been able to accomplish this without cooperation of universities such as the University of Alaska-Anchorage and the University of Wyoming in Laramie. It truly has been an enduring and effective partnership.

The above summarizes the accomplishments of WWAMI. Now let me focus on some of the challenges we face in preparing the future rural health workforce.

Over the course of the past 5 years, WWAMI has seen a drop in student interest in selecting residencies in primary care. We have gone in 1996 from approximately 36 percent of students entering into family practice to approximately 12 percent estimated this year. This remarkable decline has resulted from a variety of factors including rising student debt, student interest in assuring that there will be adequate time for personal as well as professional pursuits and changes in the healthcare delivery system. As we look to the future, the effect of this decline in student interest in primary care will be devastating for rural and medically underserved communities.

Looking deeper into the underlying reasons as to why this drop has occurred, we cite the following issues:

• *Reduced student interest in primary care.*—Long hours, limited pay, and reduced personal time have discouraged students from pursuing careers in primary care. There is frustration among many students that the current healthcare delivery system does not allow the students, once they become doctors, to pursue the principals of primary care, which include continuous patient-centered, comprehensive, compassionate, and coordinated care. The prevailing practice of primary care at the present time also discourages students away from primary care because of the limited time and infrastructure upon which to implement exceptional management of chronic diseases. This is of particular concern with an aging population and the increased incidence of chronic disease among the elderly population. Contributing to this reduction in student interest is also the increasing requirement for more positions in the current healthcare delivery system in the United States. The Association of American Medical Colleges now recommends that there be a 30 percent increase across the country in the number of medical students we train. With this increased demand, students now have many other options in healthcare that allow them to direct their interests away from primary care.

• *Increasing Student Debt.*—Over the past decade there has been a remarkable increase in student debt upon graduation from medical school. The national average is currently $125,000 per student from public schools, and $150,000+ from private schools. Students in WWAMI from Alaska currently graduate with $94,000 debt per student, with 100 percent of graduating students incurring debt. Over the past 6 years, this is up from $50,000 per student with approximately 75 percent of students graduating with debt.

• *Loss of Federal funding at the University of Washington School of Medicine/WWAMI.*—The following factors have contributed to undermining of support for our programs that are aimed at enhancing student interest in careers in primary care.

  • *Loss of title VII funding.* This loss has led to cuts in residency training in programs in Alaska and Wyoming, reduced support of Family Medicine Student Training Programs, the loss of residency faculty development fellowships, and reduced support for the underserved pathway within WWAMI.

  • *Loss of the Health Careers Opportunity Program (HCOP) Grant funding ($1.2 million over 2 years) at the University of Washington.* This has led to a severe reduction in our summer UDOC Program which is designed to encourage students from medically underserved areas to follow their interests in health careers.

  • *Loss of Center of Excellence for Native American and Native Alaskan funding.* Over the past 2 years, $647,000 has been cut from this program. At the present time, three WWAMI graduates from this program are residents at the Anchorage Family Practice Residency Program, an affiliate of the University of Washington Family Practice Network. A similar loss in Center of Excellence funding in Montana occurred in Pharmacy.

  • *Loss of funding for the WWAMI Center for Health Workforce studies and the Rural Health Research Center.* These programs fund the creation of vital sources of information (across WWAMI and the Nation) concerning the programmatic effectiveness in rural programs. In addition, they inform us concerning workforce needs in rural areas. Funding here has been reduced in the last 2 years from approximately $2 million per year to $0.6 million per year. This has resulted in our staff declining from 21 researchers to six within our Department of Family Medicine.

  • *Reduction of support for National Health Service Core Scholarships.*

• *The creation of caps on Graduate Medical Education (GME) funding as a result of the Balanced Budget Act of 1996.*—This has imposed a freeze on GME positions within the WWAMI area. Across the five States, the number of GME positions per 100,000 population is far below the Nation's average per State of 34 positions per 100,000 population. In WWAMI, this number is closer to 15 positions per 100,000. Currently the State of Alaska has only 4 residency positions per 100,000.

• *Perpetuations of GME losses currently proposed in the President's fiscal year 2008 budget.*

  • Medicare IME (Indirect Medical Education) payment reduction, a proposed cut from the GME payments that are attached to the Medicare Advantage Plan payments. There is also a potential proposed cut (as recommended by

MedPac) of an 18 percent reduction in the IME portion going from 5.5 percent to 4.5 percent.

- Proposed Medicaid cuts, including the elimination of GME payments currently provided within Medicaid payments to hospitals. If this is allowed to occur, the anticipated impact will be a loss across the country of $1.76 billion over the next 5 years.
- Nearly complete elimination of title VII—The President has proposed that title VII funding be reduced from $185 million in fiscal year 2007 to $10 million in fiscal year 2008. This is a perpetuation of significant reductions in title VII over the past 6 years.
- Reduced support for payoff of student debt by reduction of funding for the National Health Service Core from $125 million in fiscal year 2007 to $116 million in fiscal year 2008.
- Children's Graduate Medical Education appropriation reduction from $297 million to $110 million (a 63 percent reduction).

All of these reductions (and proposed reductions) have significantly influenced the ability of WWAMI and other similar programs across the country to continue to support the preparation and training of physicians to practice in rural and medically underserved areas and to achieve our remarkable outcome record. To successfully turn this around, interventions will be required in which we enhance student interest in primary care and support the continuation and expansion of programs like WWAMI.

I would strongly recommend that this committee consider support of the following Federal initiatives as a way to restore efforts on the part of programs such as WWAMI. This will assist us in continuing to provide effective medical education programs that are consistent with the workforce needs within the five States, and across the Nation.

Specifically, I would recommend the following measures be considered and taken:

- *Address the reduction in student interest and create financial incentives to entering primary care residencies and practice.* To successfully do this over time, the reimbursement for primary care physicians and physician practices will need to be enhanced far above where it is today. This reimbursement and support for primary care practices (such as the institution of measures to create medical homes for all patients, electronic medical records, and the establishment of evidence-based approaches to disease management among others) will need to occur. Specifically,

    - Encourage the increased number of medical students in training by increasing the Nation's medical school capacity consistent with the AAMC's recommendation of a 30 percent increase. Within the WWAMI States, we are currently anticipating an increase of 22 percent in seats for medical students over the course of the next 2 years. This includes 10 additional seats from the State of Alaska, 6 seats from the State of Wyoming, and 20 seats within the State of Washington. In addition, discussions of increases in seats for medical students are currently underway in Montana, and to a lesser degree in Idaho.
    - Encourage students to enter primary care residencies through tuition support programs like the National Health Service Core to offset the increasing amount of student debt, and to reduce financial disincentives to entering into primary care.
    - Restore Federal support for educational programs for physicians in training, giving particular attention to those programs that address the shortage of doctors in rural and medically underserved areas. This can be best done by restoration of title VII, HCOP and Center of Excellence Funding. We should also direct assistance to medical schools and residency training programs that promote (and are held accountable for) physicians entering practices in primary care and other needed specialties (such as general surgery and psychiatry) particularly in medically underserved areas.
    - Eliminate caps within the Medicare Program for primary care residency positions and rural track programs in specialties needed in rural America. Besides family medicine, general internal medicine and general pediatrics, this should also include innovative programs in rural track training in general surgery and in psychiatry. Many of these programs may be urban-based in addition to having rural locations in the program.
    - Expand training opportunities in rural and medically underserved communities. This should include the support for graduate medical education programs which combine urban and rural training (such as in rural track training). Enhance the supply of future accountable rural practitioners and in-

crease access to rural and medically underserved citizens to top quality healthcare. Current examples of this in WWAMI include:

1. The continuation of rural track training with the WWAMI Family Medicine Network.

2. The development (currently being considered) for rural track training in general surgery.

3. Support for rural-track psychiatry programs such as our programs based in eastern Washington, Idaho and Wyoming. This last example is of particular importance given the burgeoning problems in mental health, including meeting the needs of veterans who have returned from National Guard duty to rural communities over the past 10 years.

• *Continued support for Area Health Education Center (AHEC) funding and programs that promote recruitment of high school students into health careers.*—Programs such as the AHEC currently in place within WWAMI provide infrastructure and allow physicians in training to do community-based rotations in rural and medically underserved areas. This support needs to continue.

• *Encourage programs that promote educational relationships between Community Health Centers (CHCs) and academic medical centers.*—Within WWAMI we are currently exploring community academic linkages that would allow for increased educational opportunities within CHCs that serve rural and medically underserved populations. CHCs are rapidly becoming the greatest provider of primary care in rural and underserved urban communities, yet the supply of physicians to meet this need is far below demand. This would allow for greater opportunities to train students and residents within CHCs, and would help to alleviate the workforce shortages that challenge the CHCs.

• *Restore funding for the Office of Rural Health Policy, Rural Health Research Centers and the Bureau of Health Profession Centers for Health Workforce Study across the country.*—The absence of funding for these programs has severely limited our ability to evaluate and assess efforts that are currently in place to craft innovations that address many of the needs that I have addressed today. In addition, funding for the Nation's Centers for Health Workforce Studies (CHWS) (which has been completely eliminated within the Bureau of Health Professions) needs to be restored such that regions can have at hand the ability to assess current workforce needs.

In conclusion, it has been my privilege to present this information to you today and to provide, in a short period of time, advice to policymakers and leaders as to how we might best face the future challenges of providing for physician needs within rural and medically underserved communities. The University of Washington School of Medicine and WWAMI have long appreciated the support provided by the 10 U.S. Senators serving our five-State region, along with your colleagues from the House of Representatives. WWAMI stands ready to build upon this remarkable partnership. We will need your continued help and support in order to accomplish this task.

I look forward to answering questions that you might have around specific issues. I pledge to you to continue to provide support to this committee and your staff as we move ahead in the Federal agenda to support educational solutions to future workforce needs within the United States.

Thank you for your attention.

Senator MURKOWSKI. Thank you, Doctor, and I appreciate you making the introduction of the young men and women who are involved in the program now. It's a delight to have you here. I hope you're hearing the message that we need you.

And with that, let's go to Karen Perdue, the Associate Vice-President for Health at the University of Alaska, who has been coordinating the Task Force Report. And, I would like to note that a full copy of the Task Force Report will be included as part of the committee record.

So, with that, Ms. Perdue.

STATEMENT OF KAREN PERDUE, ASSOCIATE VICE PRESIDENT FOR HEALTH, UNIVERSITY OF ALASKA, ANCHORAGE, ALASKA

Ms. PERDUE. Thank you, Senator Murkowski. Again, I echo the appreciation that you have, the attention that you've given to this issue. Not only today, but in the last couple of years.

What I want to say, and I want to be brief, myself, because I do know that we need to have a dialogue, but Alaska has always had a physician shortage. I think those of us who have grown up here know that this is not a new phenomenon that we are facing.

So, the question that we were interested in, at the University of Alaska, in partnership with the State Health Department was, what's changed? Why is this—why are patients—anecdotally, we heard so much more access problems—has there been a change in the reimbursement climate? Are expectations of consumers higher? Do we have fewer physicians overall? The solutions for all of these things are quite expensive. The public investments that are needed for correcting the problems are expensive. So, I think it's been important to take the time to study the issue, and to give policy-makers such as yourself, verifiable information that you can rely on. And, I do believe this Report does do that.

The Report—the Task Force was appointed by the President of the University, and the Commissioner of the State, of our State Health Department. Half of the people on it were physicians, and half were not. And I think that was important, because we all came with our own questions, and our own sets of information.

We spent half of our time looking at the numbers, because—believe it or not—it's not that easy to determine how many physicians we actually have in our State, given the fact that we have many physicians who are retired, or who aren't actively practicing, this question of the military has been brought up—you know, so how many people are actually caring for patients?

I think the conclusion of the Task Force was—by the way that number was about 1,343 physicians was what we determined were practicing. I think the determination of the Task Force was that we do have a shortage. Frankly, the shortage wasn't as great as many of us expected, numerically, when we walked in the door. But, we are going to have a growing shortage, and that, I think, was the revelation of the Task Force that was probably most compelling. If we do nothing, if we do not act in a very aggressive way, we will have a growing crisis.

It is expensive to do nothing. We have learned from reports that we saw that—and we've heard earlier, over $24 million in costs are borne by our healthcare system, just the ones we're able to document—in recruiting temporary workers, and in the cost of recruitment and vacancy. One hundred and twenty five thousand dollars is spent to replace a physician in our State. Those are costs, those are funds that could be going into the remedies for the shortage, if we could just get ahead of the game.

So, the Physician Supply Task Force, of course, concluded that we needed immediate action, but probably—to reach an adequate supply by 2025, which was the planning horizon we used—that we would have to add a net of 59 physicians a year. Now, that doesn't seem like much when you look at the number, but it has to be every year. Each year, until 2025. This is a 50 percent increase in what we are gaining now.

So, what do we need to do? We need a sustained and strategic set of actions, and there's no one thing that will solve this problem, and that is, of course, a very complicated thing in public policy, because I think it's a tendency to look at a problem, address it in one way, and then say, "OK, I've got to go on to another issue." And, I say to our legislature, State legislature and our policymakers—this is not a short-term assignment that we're taking on. It's a very big job.

So, we recommended policies in four areas, and we've mentioned most of them here, so I won't go over them in detail, but I will go over them, in general.

We have to increase the in-state production of our Alaskans who go to medical school. We've heard about the WWAMI Program, we looked at those numbers, we concur that that program is extremely effective, and we're very lucky to have it. We need more slots. We said that we actually wanted 30 slots, 20 slots is—going from 10 to 20 slots is what's in front of the Legislature today, but I think, in the long run, we would like to go beyond that, in the Task Force Report we mention that. I think there's a need to keep our eye on that ball, because the University of Washington faces this pressure from every State. So, we need to act with due diligence on that.

And, of course, the residency program, we looked at that, those numbers, they were very effective, and we need more residency training.

Dr. Johnston gave us quite a lot of sobering information about how hard it is to create a residency program, how many sick people you need, and how much quality assurance you must have. So, it's not going to be an easy task, and it's not going to be cheap. But, it is definitely a highly effective way, later on in medical training, to get doctors in our State.

And finally, we looked at the issue of other medical schools, because we do have Alaskans who go to other medical schools. And Dr. David Head, who was on our Task Force, was particularly interested in this question, because he went to school at the University of Arizona. We used to have, through WHICHE, an arrangement where Alaskan students could participate in a subsidized way. And we believe that that should, that kind of an arrangement should come back to our State, but we also believe it should have a service obligation. And the poor record of return, in the old days, I think was related—in our view—to the fact that we didn't have such a service obligation.

Of course, all of that's a long timeline, so simultaneously, we must be beefing up the recruitment of physicians in our State. And, we believe that there should be a centralized place in State government where recruitment of physicians is something that people do when they get up every morning. In other words, they're not actually recruiting the physicians, but they're assisting the practices, the communities, the hospitals, and perhaps the legislative bodies in making this more effective.

Legislation, such as the ones that you sponsored—the loan repayment or the tax incentives—these are also effective for that recruitment phase, once the student has finished their medical school, and we found that was very important.

Also, we have a very strong commitment to mid-levels in our State—nurse practitioners, and physicians assistants, the University of Alaska trains them, we feel that that's important to maintain and to enhance.

And, finally, the area I want to touch on, the third area, was the medical pipeline that you've mentioned. The University of Alaska is very serious in assisting in the math and the science and the interest of young people in getting into medical careers, and particularly, to become physicians.

We have—the University of Alaska, over the last 5 years, has beefed up their medical education and pipeline programs. And through title VII, we gained many different competitive grants, to work on this area. We lost $1.4 million in effort last year, when Congress defunded that title VII, those title VII programs.

These are programs out in communities helping our students, and also working on rotations, and clinical placements for students in rural settings.

We are really anxious to work with your office and your legislation to strengthen title VII funding, I think that will have a long-term effect. Alaska does now have its own AHEC, and the partners in that Area Health Education Center include the Yukon/Kuskokwim Health Corporation, the Family Practice Residency, and the Fairbanks Memorial Hospital. These are organizations that will be going out every day and working on these problems.

So, Senator Murkowski, thank you very much for hearing about the Physician Task Force Report. We do believe that this can be turned around. We do believe—we're Alaskans, so we have to believe that we can solve these problems, that it's not hopeless. But, we will have to keep our eye on the ball, and we will have to do many things at one time.

[The prepared statement of Ms. Perdue follows:]

PREPARED STATEMENT OF KAREN PERDUE

Thank you for inviting me to participate in this field hearing on the important topic of the physician shortage and its impact on access to medical care in Alaska. In my current position at the University of Alaska, I work on a daily basis to "grow our own" healthcare professionals. These professionals are needed to fill the thousands of healthcare positions vital to the health of our Alaskan communities.

Recently, I also had the pleasure to be appointed by Secretary Leavitt as a member of the National Advisory Committee on Rural Health and Human Services and in that capacity I look forward to working on a national solution to the growing crisis of the shortage of health professionals, including physicians, in rural America.

The University of Alaska is playing a critical role in meeting the workforce needs of one of Alaska's most important industries. My comments are organized into the following areas:

(1) Documenting Alaska's Health Workforce Needs
(2) Alaska's Physician Supply Task Force
(3) Expanding and Strengthening Health Workforce Programs
(4) Recommendations

DOCUMENTING ALASKA'S HEALTH WORKFORCE NEEDS

The development and maintenance of the health workforce requires resources—resources to understand needs, develop strategies, and implement programs.

Federal funding to understand the health workforce, to track fluctuations and gaps over time, has been limited, but we have accomplished some important efforts.

Over the past 5 years, the University of Alaska has successfully partnered with the Alaska Department of Health and Social Services to support some health workforce assessments. The resultant data clearly point to huge gaps in Alaska's health workforce. Demand exceeds supply in almost every health profession.

Through 2010, the U.S. Department of Labor predicts that the top 30 fastest growing jobs in the Nation will be in the field of allied health. This finding is mirrored in Alaska, where 30 percent of the jobs created in the past 5 years are in healthcare. Further, the healthcare jobs in Alaska make up 8.3 percent of the wage and salary employment, and that may continue to grow as the population ages relative to the Lower 48 and Alaska develops more comprehensive services.

The *Status of Recruitment Resources and Strategies* (SORRAS) study commissioned by the State of Alaska's Department of Health and Social Services and conducted by the Alaska Center for Rural Health at UAA (Alaska's AHEC), documented recruitment expenditures for 13 health occupations, including oral, behavioral and physical health.[1] Specific occupations included: physicians, pharmacists, physician assistants, nurse practitioners, nurses, dentists, hygienists, psychiatrists, clinical psychologists, masters-level therapists, and licensed clinical social workers.

The 2006 study documented a staggering $24 million spent by Alaska's hospitals, community health centers, and tribal health facilities in recruiting providers for their most recent fiscal year. Of that sum, $12.9 million or 54 percent is attributed to itinerant providers.

This $24 million is lost to direct patient care, driving up the cost of doing business, compromising continuity of care and forcing organizations to make decisions on the allocation of precious resources. Equally important, the salaries to itinerant providers represent an economic loss to the communities, as itinerant providers do not buy homes or otherwise invest in the local economy.

Focusing on those occupations in the study that are supported by the National Health Service Corps, we know that respondent organizations spent an average of:

- $126,782 for the recruitment of each physician (MD or DO);
- $25,655 for the recruitment of each physician assistant and nurse practitioner; and
- $35,542 for the recruitment of each dentist.

The University of Alaska is now commissioning the Alaska Center for Rural Health to conduct a statewide Health Occupations Vacancy Study, looking at vacancies for over 100 occupations in Alaska's hospitals, nursing homes, tribal health organizations, behavioral health facilities, public health nursing, school districts, medical clinics, dental clinics, pharmacies, rehabilitation (PT, OT, Speech) clinics, diagnostic imaging clinics and medical laboratories. The resultant data will inform our program planning efforts.

PHYSICIAN SUPPLY TASK FORCE

Alaska has historically experienced a shortage of physicians, but stories from patients, providers and health policy experts seemed to point to a worsening problem.

That is why in January 2006, University of Alaska President Mark Hamilton, along with Commissioner Karleen Jackson empanelled a group of experts to take the first ever comprehensive look at Alaska's physician supply. The report of the panel, issued in August 2006 paints a challenging picture of the job in front of us: to address a current and looming physician shortage in our State. If we do not act quickly, we will face an evergrowing crisis.

The Alaska Physician Supply Task Force called for immediate action to increase the supply of physicians in Alaska. In order to reach an adequate supply of physicians by 2025, Alaska needs to add a net of 59 physicians per year, every year, starting immediately. This is a 50 percent increase in new physicians.

While these numbers may seem small at first blush, they are daunting considering the following:

- It takes between 7–10 years to train a physician.
- Only 10 Alaskans a year are currently admitted to the Alaska/University of Washington Medical School Partnership known as WWAMI. The seats have not been expanded since the program's inception in 1971.
- Alaska has only one Residency program—a common tool for recruiting new physicians.
- Competition for physicians across all disciplines will increase as shortages occur across the Nation.

---

[1] *http://nursing.uaa.alaska.edu/acrh/projects/report_sorras-05-06.pdf.*

Sustained and strategic action is needed to meet the growing shortage of physicians. No one strategy will meet the need. The Task Force recommended improvements in four areas (selected strategies listed):

(1) Increase the in-state production of physicians by increasing medical school slots and graduate medical education opportunities in Alaska.

- Increase State-subsidized medical school positions through WWAMI.
- Support and enhance residency training in Alaska.
- Support, with service obligation, Alaskans attending other medical schools.

(2) Increase recruitment of physicians.

- Create a statewide entity with resources to help communities with recruitment.
- Provide recruitment incentives like loan repayment and tax incentives to physicians who practice in rural communities.

(3) Expand and support programs that prepare students for medical careers.

- Support college prep programs in math and science, internships, scholarships.
- Support Alaska's AHEC, which is a system devoted to attracting and retaining Alaskans into health careers.

(4) Increase the retention of physicians by improving the practice environment.

- Practice environment index.

EXPANDING AND STRENGTHENING HEALTH WORKFORCE PROGRAMS [2]

The University of Alaska recognizes the growing demand for health careers academic programs and continues to innovate to make programs available throughout Alaska, and in communities where people reside.

Growing Enrollments: In the last 5 years, enrollment in health programs at the University of Alaska increased by 66 percent and the number of our graduates has grown by 55 percent.

Expansion of Distance Education: Training Alaskans in their communities for Alaska's thousands of good healthcare jobs is the only long-term solution to shortage. However, until recently, Alaska's vast geography has been a barrier to the creation of learning cohorts. That changed in 2004 with the formation of the Health Distance Education Partnership.

In its first 3 years of operation, the Health Distance Education Partnership has created over 50 distance-delivered courses covering eight occupational areas, serving over 1,000 students. Distance is not a barrier to learning. It is the future of its delivery.

National exams show that students taught by distance in nursing perform equal or out perform their own campus peers.

Doubled Nursing Supply: In 2002, the University/Industry Task Force established the goal of doubling the number of basic nursing graduates (AAS and BS programs) from the UAA School of Nursing by 2006. This goal has been met and exceeded, growing from an annual graduation of 96 to 215 students. Industry partners have given more than $4 million so far to support the expansion. Further, those industry partners also provide clinical rotation space in their hospitals. Nursing education is available in 11 Alaskan communities, enabling students to learn in the communities where they live.

Alaska WWAMI Program Expansion: Alaska WWAMI students are able to spend 3 of their 4 years of medical school in Alaska. This corresponds with the validated research that people practice where they are trained. The University of Alaska strongly supports the expansion of the Alaska WWAMI program, expansion from 10 to 20 first-year students in the coming year. The Legislature is currently considering this expansion.

Strengthening Mid-level Academic Programs: Alaska has and should maintain a higher ratio of mid-level providers (advanced nurse practioners and physicians assistants) to physicians than the national average. The University of Alaska offers Nurse Practitioner education through the School of Nursing and a Physicians Assistant Completion Program in collaboration with the University of Washington's MEDEX Northwest Physician Assistant Program. These programs should be strengthened and supported.

Alaska Area Health Education Center (AHEC) Program: Because Alaska does not have a stand alone medical school, in September 2005, Alaska's School of Nursing became the first in the Nation to have an Area Health Education Center (AHEC). All other AHEC programs in the country are housed in Schools of Medicine. Funded

---

[2] *University of Alaska Health Programs: Pathways to Alaska Health Careers.*

by the DHHS Health Resources and Services Administration,[3] the program is responsible for strengthening the health workforce via collaborations with regional partners, called AHEC Centers.

The Alaska AHEC supports strengthening the physician workforce, and does so with the following activities:

• Support of a summer program encouraging high school youth into medicine and other fields;
• Support of the WWAMI R/UOP Program, a summer experiential rotation for first year medical students;
• Support of clinical rotations for medical students throughout Alaska;
• Representation of the UW WWAMI Medical School on the AHEC Board of Directors; and
• Alaska Family Practice Residency serves as a host institution for the South Central AHEC Center.
• Fairbanks Memorial Hospital and the Yukon Kuskokwim Health Corporation also house AHEC centers.

RECOMMENDATIONS

The Federal Government has a critical role to play in addressing the physician supply issue. We make the following additional recommendations:

First, we applaud Senator Murkowski's Physician Shortage Elimination Act, which proposes to:

• Double funding to the National Health Service Corps;
• Expand current medical residency programs;
• Reauthorizes some title VII programs; and
• Bolster Community Health Centers.

Second, we strongly support the preservation of AHEC funding and other relevant Federal programs under title VII.

The University of Alaska system is severely hampered in its efforts to improve the volume and distribution of health workers due to Federal cuts that occurred in fiscal year 2006 and are being sustained in fiscal year 2007. Broadly referred to as Title VII of the Public Health Service Act, and housed in DHHS Health Resources and Services Administration's Bureau of Health Professions, these competitively awarded grants to the University of Alaska are collectively valued at $1.4 million per year and included:

• *Geriatric Education Centers,* to train physicians and other health workers in the provision of geriatric care;
• *Health Careers Opportunities Program,* to expose youth from disadvantaged backgrounds to careers in medicine and other health fields;
• *Health Education and Training Centers*, to expose village high school students to careers in health, including medicine; and
• *Quentin Burdick Rural Interdisciplinary Training*, to support interdisciplinary clinical rotations in geriatrics and behavioral health.

All these efforts came to a halt when Congress defunded large parts of title VII last year.

Alaska's AHEC provides a golden opportunity to build a statewide system of programs that work on the ground to recruit, train and retain Alaskans into health careers. Funds for this program should be enhanced.

Third, we support Federal legislation to address the rural physician shortages like the recently introduced Senate bill 498, Medicare Rural Equity Act, introduced by Senator Collins and Senator Feingold, which provides:

• Rural representation on the Medicare Payment Advisory Commission;
• Funding for quality demonstration projects in health information technology;
• Funding for hospital-based clinical rotations in underserved areas; and
• Elimination of the geographic physician work adjustment factor in the Medicare physician fee schedule.

Fourth, we recommend the U.S. Department of Labor include the health industry in list of "high growth fields."

Senator Murkowski, we look forward to working with you as you introduce the Physician Shortage Elimination Act and thank you for your leadership in addressing the physician shortage crisis in Alaska and our Nation.

---

[3] *http://bhpr.hrsa.gov/ahec/*

Senator MURKOWSKI. Thank you, Karen. You do point out the reality, for as long as most of us have been in Alaska, we've had a physician shortage issue, and it just depended on what part of the State that you were from, as to how acute it was.

But, I think we're hearing a different level of concern now. The second panel, listening to Mrs. Hatch's comments, Mr. Appel, and then Mr. Berger. The need is very immediate. And very real. When you have to make 100-plus phone calls out of the Yellow Pages to find somebody that will take your mother, we have very serious and immediate concerns that we must address.

In listening to the very distinguished panel we have here in front of us, we recognize that so many of these solutions are long-term solutions. We talk about the need to grow our own, and Dr. Johnston, I so appreciate what the residency program is doing, Dr. Coombs, what we're able to take advantage of with the WWAMI Program. But, we recognize that, for these young people, from the time that they've indicated an interest in going into medicine, and going into a program, it's going to be a few years before we're going to see them working for any of you.

So, the first question that I would throw out to those of you practicing, currently, or the others—how do we make sure that Mr. Berger finds a physician? And I know, I appreciate there are no easy answers, there's no one single solution, but let's, for discussion purposes at this moment, talk to the short-term. Is there anything that we can do for the short-term, while we work harder for the long-term solutions to do more about growing our own? Mr. Tanner, Mr. Neubauer, Mr. Perkins, anybody have any good short-term solutions?

Dr. TANNER. I came to Alaska 2 years ago after an inability to sustain a practice in the State of Washington. So, a lot of the people have been here a long time, I'm relatively new to the State, I got nominated to—as President of the Alaska State Medical Association—things develop very quickly.

My experience within, as a general internists—I specialize primarily in the field of diabetology, and also lipidology, which is preventative cardiology, basically, there's not really a defined specialty within that. But, the complexity of the patients that I see everyday, it's very time-consuming.

In order to make a practice work in the State of Alaska, you'd have to average seeing a patient every 7 minutes. I can't say "hello" in 7 minutes, let alone, review medications, and "Oh, by the way," you know, you've got multiple problems.

In 1 year, before I got here, with my mother being my receptionist, my wife being my office manager, and being very efficient at managing my office, in 1 year, my net income was nothing. It's hard to believe that I could make more money working at Chuck E. Cheese, than I could actually operating in a practice. There's a conflict between the doctor and the patient—that the doctor and patient are being thrown into, in that in some way we're looking like the bad guys—that we're not accepting patients. And in any trade, when you increase the cost of doing business—my receptionist needs benefits, my office manager now needs to have a salary for her children. My nurse needs to have a salary—as everything is going up and reimbursements are going down, what that means is, you need to see more and more patients, and that time—the valuable time that you spend with your doctor where you sit down and analyze what is exactly going on—is going out the window.

So, in order for me to stay financially soluble, I need to be paid for what I do—just like the electrician, just like the plumber, just like anybody that has a trade that they offer.

And so, as the reimbursements continue to go down, and continue to be threatened to be cut even further, it's going to get worse. And, you just have to pay for what you're getting, and there's a value to things and goods that are delivered in other professions, but this is a right that everybody should have, is going to the doctor. And, I'm with the fellow from the western part of the State, in Bethel, in saying you need to have that continuity, that's why I went into internal medicine.

I actually was groomed, you know, when I was going through my program, "Oh, you're really, you know, you're a good doctor, we want you to be a cardiologist, we want you to be a gastroentologist," always this push to be a sub-specialist. No, I want to be a general internist. I like the continuity of knowing patients over a number of years. But, you do get disincentivized because you're not being paid. And then you hear a lot of doctors that are upset, and daily focus on this. And it's like, you know, I do have the best job in the world. To sit down with a patient and make a difference in their lives and saying, if I have the time—and it's not a narcissistic thing—I can prevent you from having many devastating things happen in your life.

And it impacts other things, I talked to a fellow coming back from Washington, DC., when I saw you, he's over 65 years of age, and I say, "What do you do for a doctor?" And he goes, "I just go to the emergency room." I mean, that is not an appropriate way of handling—but he says he has no choice.

So, the money's being spent elsewhere, when really, the money should be spent with the primary care doctors. And, I'm the cheapest thing that Medicare can spend their money on. Labs are very expensive. One hour with a cardiologist, doing a procedure—extremely expensive. Going to the emergency room—extremely expensive. But, the total cost for me, in a year, is probably less than $500, and I can prevent a lot of those things from happening.

So, that's how you immediately can fix it—is we have to be paid. And, it's not a greed thing, I don't have a bunch of money in a room, I just go run into and jump in every day——

[Laughter.]

Dr. TANNER [continuing]. It is a problem of being able to keep the doors open to my practice because i can't pay everybody, and then the bureaucracy that goes along with insurance companies, and getting things authorized and those things—it takes staff, just to get things authorized through an insurance company. My authorization should be me signing my name on a prescription, that's my authorization.

Senator MURKOWSKI. You point out that a doctor has the—certainly the right to be compensated, just as an electrician or a plumber, and I don't think that if a plumber were to have expenses of 100 percent, he would accept compensation at 40 percent, and yet that's what we're asking of those docs who do see the Medicare patients.

Dr. Neubauer, do you want to jump in? Short-term solutions.

Dr. NEUBAUER. Yeah, I think that partly the answer depends on what your definition of short-term is. If you mean, in the next couple of years, I think it's likely that things are going to get worse before they get better. Because there's—it's almost like a perfect storm right now—the capacity in private practice, to add new physicians here who do what I do, is very limited. And partly that is because general internists in this town have—as a rule—pared down their practices to bare bones. You know, they work in small offices that have very little capacity to add another physician, and they've pared down their expenses, in an effort to survive, so that they can keep going.

So, the surge capacity in the private world is very limited right now.

You know, I think that in the sort of longer short-term, there's more hope. And that is that I think there's a lot of willingness on the part of young people coming up and training to do the work. I'd be interested in what the students here would say, but I think the attractiveness of being a doctor—I mean, you know, seeing patients, thinking, trying to solve their problems—is great. And the push to go into fields of medicine that are highly technical, highly compensated, is primarily a financial one.

I think there would be a much more even spread of what people went into, if there weren't these gigantic differences in what a highly paid technical physician makes, versus somebody who does what I do, and what Dr. Tanner does, which is sit in an office and think. You know, it's a lot of fun to think, and it does a lot of good, and I think there's a lot of attractiveness to it. It's a different kind of work than reading an echocardiogram, or sitting and reading x-rays all day—which is also very important. But, I think there needs to be a bigger spread of what people go into. And right now, there's a tremendous push to go into the higher paid things.

One thing that I think needs to happen is for there to be a continuity of things, that when a physician leaves practice, that somebody else wants to come and do their work and take it over, not just have it end. And that, unfortunately, has been the model here, as I mentioned in my testimony. It's a huge tragedy, when I see a physician retire here, and, as I said, close their doors, charts go in storage, patients scattered to the wind. That's absolutely wrong. There should be a willingness of somebody young to come and take on that practice, and right now, there's just no incentive to do that. It's not looked at as something of value.

And I can cite to you example after example of physicians who have left here over the last 25 years I've been observing and that that has happened. It's an extreme tragedy.

Senator MURKOWSKI. Let's just focus on the recruitment issue for a second, because that's—as you point out, an area where we're not able to provide for the continuity of care that I think we would all like to see. When you have somebody who's retired, or you've got an expanding medical practice, and you've got room to take on more, if you could find the physician to come in.

I understand that here in Anchorage, where we've got our only rheumatologist in the State, we've got one rheumatologist who's been trying to retire for years, but he can't do it because there's nobody who will step up and take his practice, and his commitment to his practice is such that he doesn't want to leave them in the lurch.

But, yet at some point in time you've got to have that backfill, if you will, you've got to have those reinforcements to step up.

When we did the Town Hall meetings last year, the stories that I was hearing about the medical practices that had been looking for 18 months to fill a slot for an internist, 2 years to fill a slot for an internist—what else are we doing wrong that we can't attract them?

Part of it, as I recall, was the great lure of coming to Alaska, and the adventure of being here. But, I guess the adventure of being in Alaska, is outweighed by the fact that you might not be able to afford your Alaskan adventure, is that still our situation?

Dr. NEUBAUER. Well, you know, I think more money is always good.

Senator MURKOWSKI. Money always helps.

[Laughter.]

Dr. NEUBAUER. And I think that is one solution, honestly. But, I think there are a few others. I think that Electronic Health Records have great promise. I think that if an office has a robust Electronic Health Record, that's a saleable point for somebody coming in, wanting that practice. And, I think in general, across the country, it's almost expected for young physicians, the few that are going into primary care practices right now, to want that and have it as a requirement.

So, I think that's very important. And, that's something that, I mean, this is a wealthy State, we should be supporting physicians in ways that we can, by giving them subsidies to put in place Electronic Health Records, and I mean the physicians who are in practice now. Because I think that would not only be a recruitment point, but also something that would make it much more likely that when they leave practice, that somebody would be there to take their place.

So, more money, and Electronic Health Records, that would be a good start. And, I think, increasing the pipeline of people coming in is extremely important. I mean, if there's nobody interested in taking the job, you're sunk in the water. So, you have to have people coming up in the pipeline who want to be there.

But, then you have to incentivize for them to want to do that, and be able to do that. Because, I think, when you're saddled with $150,000 to $300,000 of debt, you're not going to do what I do for a living. It's, you've already bought two houses before you're going into practice.

Senator MURKOWSKI. Dr. Coombs.

Dr. COOMBS. Well, I'd like to make a couple of comments. First of all, I think we've heard from the panel, but also I think the students in the audience would agree that they are going into medicine because of the fact that they want to make a difference. That they are very happy with a professional life and the kinds of things that they can do for others, that's not the issue.

I think the issue is dealing with the stark realities that we enter into, in terms of both—two things. First of all, once you have a shortage of people, then you never have enough to be able to meet the needs, and that is something that preys upon your private life, in addition to your professional life. Especially in isolated, small communities.

The second thing is, dollars. Fund it, and they will come. If you look at, as an example, two things that I'll give you an example of—in Washington State where I practice, currently private insurance pays up about $56 per relative value unit to take care of a patient. Medicare pays about $36. Medicaid pays about $22. It's impossible to meet the overheads, which are now 60 to 70 percent in a primary care office, to be able to provide for just the care that you have to provide, and the staff that you have to provide to achieve that.

In addition to that, you have debt, and other considerations. So, the unfortunate thing, is that students and many professionals now run into the stark reality, which is something where they have to do something which really is survival mode, in terms of the ability to keep the door open, to allow patients to come in the door. And that means, restricting the patients that they see.

It's not something that's part of the Hippocratic Oath. It is not something that we went into medicine to do. It's just reality.

Senator MURKOWSKI. I'm going to go a little out of line here, a little unorthodox for a hearing, but I'm going to ask some of you students who are part of the WWAMI Program, what would incentivize you to stay here in the State, to go into the areas of— as Dr. Neubauer has indicated—into the primary care, internist areas? What's it going to take to keep you here, to provide the level of service that we would like to see for Alaskans? And, if I can just ask you to stand if you want to share a thought with us, and speak loudly so that we can pick you up on record.

What have we got? Probably better if you could come up to the mike; you don't even need to get fancy.

MELISSA. My name's Melissa, and part of it for me is, you know, I'm facing $100,000 of debt, and that's really scary. I want to know that I'm going to be able to, you know, pay that back. And, for me, it does come down to money, and being able to deal with my loans, and sort of having help with assisting that, and incentive programs to come back here.

Senator MURKOWSKI. Where are you from, Melissa?

MELISSA. I'm from Eagle River.

Senator MURKOWSKI. We want you to come back.

MELISSA. I want to come back. I mean, Alaska is a great place to grow up, so I'd love to come back here, so hopefully it will work out.

Senator MURKOWSKI. OK, we'll work on that.

Who else has a—what would allow you to continue to stay here in Alaska?

ROSS BALDWIN. Ross Baldwin from Kenai, Alaska.

I'm actually not too concerned about the whole debt thing, because I'm interested in surgery, and I'm going to get a lot of dirty looks right now.

But, one thing that does concern me, as these guys addressed over here, and I actually got to spend some time working under Dr. Perkins—he's an amazing guy—but, the lack of residency programs in the State, or that feed into residency programs in the State, is a huge concern for me.

If I want to do a surgical residency, which is roughly 7 years, 6 or 7 years from my understanding—I can't be in Alaska for those 6 or 7 years. So——

Senator MURKOWSKI. So, 7 years, you're gone.

ROSS BALDWIN. Right.

Senator MURKOWSKI. What happens if you fall in love with somebody who doesn't want to come back to Alaska? What do we do to make sure that we can have residency programs for somebody like you?

ROSS BALDWIN. I don't have any excellent solutions, because I don't have enough knowledge about residency programs at this point.

[Laughter.]

Senator MURKOWSKI. Then we're just going to have to hope that you find a young woman here.

ROSS BALDWIN. Right.

Part of the problem is that we have a small population base, and a lot of the surgical residencies are uncomfortable with putting forward a residency program with that small patient base.

I think that there's some innovative solutions out there, I'm not qualified to offer any of those, but I definitely think that there could be something done to increase residencies, not just in the surgical area, but beyond basic family practice. Internist residency, I think, would be an excellent addition to the State.

And also, just to kind of give you some additional perspective from our community. I grew up in Kenai, and I went to a clinic there where there was a primary care physician, and he just closed his doors, and there's no one coming in to replace him. The need is real, it's very, very real.

So, thank you for your time.

Senator MURKOWSKI. Thank you, Ross.

The statistics that we have out there are so troubling, though, when you recognize that the majority will stay in practice, what is it, within 100 miles of where they have done their residency. So, that just automatically precludes so many of the young Alaskans, if you're going to go outside for 6 or 7 years to do that residency.

What do we do, Dr. Johnston?

Dr. JOHNSTON. Well, I think there's, really logically, only a couple things that can be done. The range of possibilities is not huge. We can have residencies here in Alaska, or we can have branches of residencies here in Alaska. And, really, those are about the only two ways that you're going to have that final phase of graduate training in the State.

The data that you cited that depends on specialty a little bit— but around 70 percent of residency graduates practice within 100 or 150 miles of where they train—are based upon graduates of full-fledged residencies, where the resident does their whole 3 years in that program, such as our program here in Alaska.

There are other possibilities where residencies in other States, such as Washington, could have residents rotate in Alaska for a period of time, as a way for us to make them fall in love with the State, so that after they graduate from their residency in Washington they would want to come up here and practice. I don't know that there's any data on how effective that is in attracting people to ultimately practice in the State, maybe Dr. Coombs knows more, because he's involved with graduate medical education on a larger scale than I am.

But the University of Washington, WWAMI program has proposed to us, on several occasions, to try to develop those kinds of programs with the idea that it would allow Alaskans an opportunity to do at least some of their surgical residency here in their home State. If that's going to keep them from falling in love with a woman from Washington, I don't know. But, maybe we can have a parade of young ladies there that——

[Laughter.]

Senator MURKOWSKI. That's not going to be part of our medical solution.

Dr. Coombs.

Dr. COOMBS. I'd just like to make a comment on Dr. Johnston's— I was in Boise, Idaho last week, and we were just establishing a psychiatry residency, actually, in Idaho, that will be shared 2 years in Seattle, 2 years in Boise, which is a combination between the Boise V.A. and the two downtown hospitals in Boise.

We've had success, since 1991, with psychiatry residency like that model in Spokane, and I know Senator Murray is on your committee, where we've had 2 years Seattle, 2 years Spokane—64 percent of its graduates have gone into practice in the Greater Spokane area, 84 percent in eastern Washington. And mental health is a huge issue in that respect. I know that's something that, in Idaho, they're delighted to see that.

In general, internal medicine, we have had a program, again, in conjunction with the Boise V.A.—I mention the V.A., because the V.A. right now is in the process of increasing by almost 1,000 residency slots nationwide, in terms of increasing the amount of residency positions which are supported. I'd love to see that come to fruition here in the Greater Anchorage area, to engage the V.A. in terms of residency training.

But our internal medicine program, again, based at the Boise V.A., has been responsible, with over 80 percent of its graduates going into practice within the WWAMI area, including within the State of Idaho, 57 percent. So, those are general, internal medicine, primary care, and total medicine residents. There are models, it's a matter of having, I think, the flexibility within the GME process to be able to do that. Not only in funding, but also in the accreditation cycle.

Senator MURKOWSKI. Now, Dr. Johnston, you had mentioned that Alaska has the lowest number of students coming, of being accepted into the medical schools, if I remember that recap.

Ms. Perdue, we recognize, and our Task Force has been looking at the shortage, is—from the University perspective, should we be doing more to encourage, at the high school and the college level, the interest in getting into this healthcare pipeline? I mean, we acknowledge that we don't have a lot of folks here in the State, but our reality is that we should be doing a little bit better about growing our own, but if we don't have people that are interested in getting in that pipeline at all, it's going to be tough to achieve what many of you have suggested. Are we pursuing that, at all, through the University?

Ms. PERDUE. Well, the University, as I mentioned, has been focusing on beefing up all of its healthcare opportunities, from nursing to——

Senator MURKOWSKI. You've been very successful with the nursing component.

Ms. PERDUE. Correct. So, we find the interest is there, but we find that the need for the math skills, and the science skills and so on, you know, really must be taken care of, hopefully not after the student starts to apply for the program. In other words, there are summer opportunities, and if you can't get those programs in your high school, they can be supplemented—those are all things that many of the title VII programs that we talked about, are meant to enhance in our State. Not that that's solely the responsibility of the Federal Government—certainly the school districts and the University working together have a need for that.

Because it's not only for students going into medical careers, it's engineering, and other areas where we need those technical skills. But, we need those internships, we need those summer programs, we need that exposure for rural students, and urban students alike. And we are very anxious to do more of that.

Senator MURKOWSKI. I've got a whole host of questions, I could keep you here all afternoon, but we only have the hearing room until noon today, and we do have some additional folks that have indicated they would like a couple minutes at the microphone, so I want to give them that opportunity.

I think it was you, Dr. Tanner, who mentioned that with the recent military deployment there has been even further pressure on the local practitioners to pick up the patients of those who were being seen by some at the medical unit there at Elmendorf. Can you give me a little bit more in terms of background on that, and how it has affected the practice here in the area, and the pressures?

Dr. TANNER. What I can respond to is what happens in my office, and people calling my office daily. And it seems, we get more questions with regard to taking some of the military-sponsored insurances as they're supplemental insurances, as well as, the numbers have increased since we've seen the conflict in the Middle East. The specific numbers, I'm not sure of.

Senator MURKOWSKI. Any—Dr. Neubauer, are you getting the same inquiry?

Dr. NEUBAUER. I'm not sure. What I do know is that my office gets, probably 10 to 20 calls a day for new patients that want to come into my practice, and the others in my office, and we take some of those.

One of the things, just to mention, that I think that there's a tremendous willingness on the part of doctors to try and do the right thing. You know, I think there have been a number of doctors in

Anchorage that have opted out of Medicare altogether, and that's not healthy when you have such a small number of doctors.

Tri-Care, I'm not sure what's going on with taking Tri-Care patients right now. But, I do know that between all of the patients seeking care, there's just no way that primary care doctors who are here can do all of what needs to be done.

Senator MURKOWSKI. Do I understand correctly that, if you are going to accept Medicare patients, you basically have to opt-in or make a statement that you will be accepting those patients, and you essentially make that statement on an annual basis. And if you decide at the beginning of 2007 that you are not going to be taking any Medicare patients, you may not take any for the duration of that year?

Dr. NEUBAUER. There's three ways you can handle the Medicare program. One, is by being a participating physician, which means that when you see a Medicare patient, you can't bill the patient at all, you bill the Medicare program and are reimbursed directly from Medicare.

You can be what is called a nonparticipating physician, which is kind of a misnomer. And what that basically means is that when you see a Medicare patient you can bill the patient, and you're allowed to bill them up to the Medicare-allowable rate, which is actually a little bit more than you get if you just get paid by Medicare. And you can collect from the patient, and then the patient can collect from Medicare to be reimbursed part of that fee.

And, so it's not really nonparticipation, it's just a different kind of participation. And then you can opt-out, which means you do all the things to basically say, "I'm going to have nothing to do with the Medicare program," and then you can bill the patient whatever you want. And that's something—as I say, I think—two physicians that I know of, two internists in Anchorage have done.

That's pretty extreme, and basically, I know in my patient population, that would essentially disenfranchise most of my patients. I mean, I have a few wealthy patients who could pay, you know, huge fees if I wanted to charge them, but most of my patients are just struggling along, and so, I just, frankly, couldn't do that to them.

But, there are a few physicians who have taken that route, just kind of in disgust, I think, over what's going on.

The 40 percent number is real—I've just looked at what my charges are versus what I get from Medicare, and it's 40 percent. And, I can tell you, it's very, very difficult. I mean, we struggle on a day-to-day, month-to-month basis to just pay the bills. And I don't make an extravagant salary at all. So, it's just very difficult to run a business that way. In fact, it's getting more difficult, and it may get close to impossible, if it gets worse.

Senator MURKOWSKI. Dr. Tanner, and then I want to ask Dr. Johnston a question.

Dr. TANNER. One thing is that, there are physicians that can opt out, but the patient can't opt out. If you turn 65 years of age, you have to take Medicare as your primary unless you are full-time employed.

There are patients that would like to opt-out and use their State benefits as an insurance, to be their primary carrier, but they don't have that opportunity.

The other thing is there's a misconception amongst a lot of patients that, if they have a deductible that it pays the physician the difference between the routine fees and Medicare fees. And that's not allowed. There, it's paid at the hospital, they pay their labs, but the secondary insurance pays nothing to us. And so, just a couple things where they're, they could—actually just allowing patients to opt-out of Medicare would eliminate some patients off the Medicare roll, so to speak, and then——

[Applause.]

Dr. TANNER [continuing]. And then allowing Medicare to allow a secondary insurance to pay the difference and just those two things right there would allow the physicians, actually, to incorporate Medicare back in their practice. Because it may come close to what we normally would be paid by insured patients, but it allows a little bit more flexibility rather than just making everybody do it. Thank you.

Senator MURKOWSKI. Very good point.

Dr. Johnston, I wanted to ask you about the caps. You had mentioned that—if we were able, if we could remove those caps that are in place—were we to do so, how many new residents could we bring into the residency training program?

Dr. JOHNSTON. Well, currently our residency program is planned around having 36 residents, that's 12 per year for a 3-year program, and our cap is about 22. We can't really—we're already operating at a substantial deficit.

If the caps were lifted so that we could count all 36 of our residents, that would just about fix the biggest part of our current deficit.

The controlling factor—if there were no caps at all—the controlling factor and the size of the residency would be such things as teaching opportunities, the size of the facility where the residents practice and train, and those sorts of things.

You know, just off the top of my head without planning it, I would say our program could probably go to maybe 15 per year from the 12 that it is now, which would be a significant increase. But the interesting thing about lifting the caps, would be then it would create the opportunity for us in Alaska to start opening other residency programs. You know I have a pro forma that I'm going to be discussing about starting a psychiatry residency program here. A general internal medicine residency would be something that could easily be done in a place like Providence, because we have the quality teachers, we have the quality physicians and we have the patient base. Parts of a surgery residency could be done here in Alaska. A pediatric residency would be possible. But we can't do any of those now because residency education is so expensive, that without a funding stream to support, no institution is going to go out on a limb and start a residency program. Right now Providence Hospital, the only sponsoring institution for a residency in Alaska, is losing $2 million a year to keep our program going. They're not going to start another program that's going to lose them another $2 million a year, so they have to have a funding stream.

And so the caps—my feeling is that if our residency program as it is now or slightly larger—operates for a number of years, we will be satisfying the need for primary care, for family physicians for Alaska. Because we're the biggest residency program in the Northwest, in the WWAMI region right now. We're the biggest family medicine residency program of all the WWAMI States. But we're not going to solve the physician problem in Alaska by just pumping out more family doctors. We have to be able to produce the other specialties that are really needed in the State and we can't even touch that until we can get the caps lifted.

Senator MURKOWSKI. Well, and when we figure we need 59 new physicians a year for—through the year 2025 to just become on par with the population-to-physician ratio in the Lower 48. Even adding those additional slots, it just seems like you can't get ahead of the wave here.

Dr. TANNER. Can I comment briefly on a question you asked earlier, which is what can we do immediately to fix the problem? And the problem seems to be that there just aren't doctors out there that want to come to Alaska, and join Dr. Neubauer or the other practices that are, that would be able to recruit and have these physicians if they were around.

I think the problem is that shrinking supply nationally—and in a world of a shrinking national supply—you have to be extremely competitive in order to be able to draw the few that are available to your place as opposed to having them practice somewhere else. We're not very competitive in recruitment right now. Because the people who are trying to recruit are docs, like Dr. Neubauer who are in small offices. They don't have the resources just to keep their doors open hardly, let alone advertise, go on trips to residency programs in the other parts of the United States to solicit, pay recruitment sign-on bonuses, guarantee the salary for the first couple years, pay the recruitment trips where they come up and interview and meet the docs and everything—they don't have the resources to do that. So we're totally noncompetitive in that.

Some of the hospitals are stepping up to that plate trying to help out. Their budgets for that are very limited as well. If you want an immediate solution to the problem of physician shortage, we have to get organized and get aggressive about a recruitment process and that has to be done on a much larger scale than the individual practices. Which is one of the reasons that the Physicians Supply Task Force made a recommendation for a statewide office to help support those activities. But that's going to have to be funded, because there's a significant amount of cost that goes into those kinds of activities. And if anything can be done on the Federal level to help fund that I think that would be very beneficial.

Senator MURKOWSKI. Very constructive.

Excellent comments. I appreciate the input from each of you. It's quite apparent that there is passion at all levels, whether within your respective practice or what you're doing to cultivate those physicians who will be serving us.

But I appreciate, again, all that you have provided us with here today, in terms of your insight and the possible solutions, both long- and short-term. I thank you.

And we now will have an opportunity for individuals to make very brief comments. I'd ask that you try to limit your comments to no more than a couple minutes. And I realize you may feel that that's not fair because these folks had a good opportunity to present theirs, but I do want to be able to hear from everyone.

I do have a sign in sheet that we will follow off of. The first person that we will hear from is Diane Holmes. The second is Diane DeSanto, and then we will go to Jenna Lundy. So if those of you who are not on a list wish to testify, I would just ask that you line up there toward the back.

Ms. Holmes, welcome.

Ms. HOLMES. Senator, my comments are of course directed to you, but also if they'll stick around, to the WWAMI students.

I'm a detail person and I do have some solutions that I hope you will hear me out including how to get or keep people here, good medical people here.

There's unnecessary shortcomings to this system. The first situation I'd like to bring to your attention is that Medicare regulations actually cause higher costs. I am discouraged from getting lab work at the cheapest, but quality, lab in this town because Medicare— I can not submit Medicare forms, because my lab will not submit Medicare forms—and the regulations that might allow me to be reimbursed are beyond ridiculous.

Why can't the reimbursement procedures be streamlined so that I can submit my $35 lab fee that gives me three times the amount of tests than a somewhat similar one at the hospital? Granted, I was not a Medicare patient at the time. However, there is a page in the Medicare Web site, and I have an outdated form that should allow me to submit my claims and be reimbursed myself, but it is so ridiculous. I can not do this until 15 months have passed. There needs to be something done so that I can do this myself.

Regarding the web information, you're not the webmaster and I won't bore you with the details, but it is inaccurate, and I could do a much better job, and I hope you will put me to the right person.

Are you aware about the contracts? There are doctors in this town who require their Medicare customer to sign a contract to be seen. I'm told by my secondary insurance——and by that I mean the company, actually the State, secondary insurance that pays the paltry 20 percent of the remaining Medicare allowable fee—that if I sign a contract they will not pay that 20 percent. I don't know how they're going to find out if I have paid that or not, but, and I don't even know if I can submit to Medicare after I have paid that, but these are things that need to be looked into.

No. 3, the bill. There's a bill that the doctors could charge me 115 percent of what is allowable for a Medicare CPT code procedure. Why can't I just pay the difference between that and the regular bill, as you just heard some of the doctors say? I could get my miles and submit my own claim.

[Applause.]

I have been doing that for a long time, and as long I have the grey matter to fill out the forms, why not let me? And if by doing this, this would allow some Medicare customers to be seen by the doctors because those of us that may be able to pay the full difference, can. And we would be, then, a regular paying customer.

And the last thing I'd like to say, how do you get more doctors to stay here? I'm afraid you have to look beyond medicine. You have to look as to what makes a healthy community, and a healthy person. And that is, we want to make a livable city so that these— I call them kids, they are pretty young—will want to come back. We need a walkable city, and we have to make sure that we have a city that has good northern climate land use designs.

And it's very appropriate right now because we have title 21 coming up and this Administration and the people in Juneau can do an awful lot to making good northern city communities, particularly with the $93 million sitting there now to be given probably, unfortunately to Anchorage for a bridge to nowhere, very soon.

Senator MURKOWSKI. Thank you Ms. Holmes.

Diane Santo. Oh, okay.

Welcome Mr. Jesse.

Mr. JESSE. Thank you, Senator. Again, our appreciation for holding this hearing. Diane DeSanto, unfortunately, had to go back down to the Mayor's office.

Well, certainly this is an issue for many of us, particularly around psychiatry and particularly around children's psychiatry. Listening to the testimony about doing residencies and partial residencies, all of those opportunities I think are very positive. If we could set that sort of thing up in Alaska, particularly now with our Bring the Kids Home initiative, where we are building in-state capacity and partnership with the University on workforce issues— I think if we are able to develop that kind of a connection between those people that have these skills and are interested in serving this population—I think this could be a very positive thing. Certainly the Mental Health Trust Authority would be interested in partnering and developing that kind of residency program within the State.

So with that, good luck, and thank you very much.

Senator MURKOWSKI. Thank you, we appreciate what you do with the Mental Health Trust Authority.

Next we have Jenna Lundy, and following Jenna we have Chad Whitaker, and then Wayne Westburg.

Ms. LUNDY. Senator Murkowski, I'm really nervous, but thanks for letting me speak. I'd like to respond first of all that I do not think that there's a quick fix.

I have here a teacher orientation book from 1968 that was produced by the Bureau of Indian Affairs. My family came to Alaska at that time and let me just read for a moment, the section on village health states,

> "The teacher plays a major role in disease prevention. Good health practices are learned chiefly in the school. The teacher has an obligation to become acquainted with prevalent health problems, and methods of prevention. Medical personnel should be consulted, and practical health routines developed, which can be observed in the home as well as in school. Some common health problems: eye and ear infections, respiratory ailments, skin infections, dental cavities, stomach and intestinal disorders."

Any of you that practice medicine in this room today knows that those are the things that the people in our villages face now. So next year will mark 2008. In 40 years, this list has not changed. Forty years. Is there a quick fix?

And then this report that, actually I just browsed through while I was sitting here, but one of the other concerns that I have just from comments that were made—it says real clearly here that healthcare workers who grow up in a rural location are more likely to be recruited to rural practice. Can we, indeed, bring people from the Lower 48 to places, perhaps Anchorage, perhaps Girdwood—but can we bring someone to Bethel where I grew up? Can we bring someone to Hooper Bay? Can we bring someone to the Village of Napakiak, to Fairbanks, to Tok where I was last week, but only because I had canceled the previous trip because it was 52° below? How do we bring someone from the States to practice medicine in a place like Tok where it does, you know, reach 52° below? Anchorage is pretty mild. Homer, the Kenai—pretty mild climates.

We have trouble maintaining physicians out in rural Alaska. We don't have any, at all. The wait time is 3, 4, 6 months out before someone can see a specialist.

I recently had a very, very close friend who went to ANMC here, in Anchorage, and was not referred to a specialist, because her condition wasn't chronic. When Dr. Neubauer spoke of a person in his practice who retired, that person came to this lady's aid, and because he was willing to do—come out of retirement—that woman is alive, today, literally. He saved her life.

But, that isn't actually what I came to—what I asked to speak to today. I'm an educator by training, and so I can also relate to being paid for the services that you're providing, equitably. And I do understand that there are many physicians that go into the practice of medicine not merely because of the amount of money that they're going to make, but because of the human service that they're going to provide.

Out in the Bethel area, we are blessed with Dr. Carpenter, who is a dentist. He did fall in love with Bethel, he did fall in love with the people of the YK Delta, and he chose to stay there and serve those people.

Dr. Breneman, I'm sure that there are other doctors that could be listed, from around the State—but those people have either passed on, or they've retired. And, these young people that are sitting here—I hope that they are going to step into those shoes. When I hear of the young man that's from Kenai, I hope that he chooses to go back to practice in Kenai.

I know the allure of the States, as I keep saying, but the allure is great. And many of our retirees are leaving, also, because it's great. But, I would like to say that two of my colleagues are here with me, and we work with Head Start, and we work with an organization that has 24 Head Start programs across the State, and we have five early Head Start programs. We serve 161 children in the early Head Start program—that's birth to three. And, of those 161 children, only 64 of them are up to date on their well-child screenings. And, I have numbers and statistics that I won't go on and on about, but thank you for listening.

Senator MURKOWSKI. Thank you, I appreciate it. Thank you for giving us that rural perspective.

Jed Whitaker, followed by Wayne Westburg.

Mr. Whitaker.

Mr. WHITAKER. Thirty-one cents of every healthcare dollar goes to the paperwork and administrative costs of a healthcare system convoluted by insurance. The high cost of healthcare is due to the inefficiency and greed of the insurance industry.

You are quoted as saying we are facing a physician shortage crisis in Alaska. Your solution, like any good Republican, is to give a tax cut of $1,000 a month to doctors to entice them to service Alaska. Doctors, who are already in the highest income bracket, bribed to practice medicine in Alaska. Solid Republican rhetoric, because Republicans understand bribes.

Solid Republican rhetoric that asks us to support the war criminal in the White House, and the trillion dollar costs of fighting a war that cannot be won, fighting a people who did not attack America. Rhetoric that says, "Support the troops," with one tongue, while the other tongue cuts Veterans' benefits, and Medicare. Rhetoric that eliminates the Estate Tax, a tax which frees just one family, the Waltons, heirs of Wal-Mart, a $32 billion windfall, with one tongue, while the other tongue cuts Medicare by $28 billion. Solid Republican rhetoric that would have us believe that tax cuts for the rich are good for the country, while the cost of going to college has risen 35 percent in the last 4 years. Rhetoric that opposes a living minimum wage, let alone a minimum wage that could pay for the cost of attending medical school. Solid Republican rhetoric that equates military might with national security, while the health of Americans—the real national security—fails.

The annual cost of the war in Iraq is approximately $120 billion a year. Supplemented by sole-source contracts, to Christian right private army corporations, like Blackwater, and friends of Cheney, like Halliburton, who approach a total cost, to date, of close to a trillion dollars. A trillion dollars to fight a war that cannot be won, killing a people who did not attack America. That $120 trillion a year could pay for universal healthcare, for all Americans, not just Alaskans. It could also pay for a free college education, and the cost of medical school for at least two—if not more—people from every village and city in Alaska.

If you are really serious about solving a physician shortage crisis in Alaska, stop funding the War in Iraq, and start funding a program to help the people of Alaska become doctors.

To have this hearing today, you did not do your job. There was a nonbinding resolution opposing the escalation of the War in Iraq. You didn't even—you weren't even there to vote, to allow that debate to continue. Shame on you.

That is the reason why we have a shortage. We are not investing in our people. Instead, we are conducting wars that are illegal and immoral all across this world at a tremendous cost. Giving tax cuts to the rich, and creating big budget deficits. And now, with the Democrats pay-go, all the ideas that were presented to you by all of the esteemed panelists cannot be funded—cannot be funded—because the Democrats are going to insist that the budget be balanced. And the only way that you're going to be able to balance that budget, is to end the War in Iraq.

Senator MURKOWSKI. Thank you, Mr. Whitaker.

Mr. Wayne Westburg.

WAYNE WESTBURG. Thank you for being here, Senator.

I'm 68 years old, and I work full-time, and I've, in the last 6 months, had an interesting education. My doctor in—and I'm sorry, some of this is redundant, but I think it's worth emphasizing—my doctor informed me he was retiring. Consequently, I've spent about the last 6 months calling clinics, doctors all around town, and have found that nobody—virtually nobody—is taking new Medicare patients.

And, I don't believe it's because of the workload. Being the individual that I am, I got into some intense questioning of office personnel and that—I never really did get through to talk to a doctor—and the reason that they're unable to accommodate new Medicare patients is pure and simple, money. That, and a second issue is paperwork, and the bureaucratic hassle of trying to collect from Medicare, which apparently is quite a problem, also.

I even offered, naively, to pay the difference. I feel that's a right that we should have, and they can't legally accept any additional payment for Medicare-reimbursed services.

Interestingly, I just had a colonoscopy, and I had no problem finding a specialist to do it, who would handle, who would take Medicare. I'm in the process of shopping for new knees, and I have no problem coming up with specialists to do that stuff. It would appear that the problem is Medicare payment on general practitioners. And, I hesitate to use the term discriminatory—I don't know if it's purposeful, but for some reason, they're just not reimbursing the GPs what they need, and the constant statement is, "It doesn't even cover our overhead."

Now, I have actually come up with a solution to the problem, and it may be one that more and more seniors are going to have to take, and that is, I've gotten with a nurse provider. And I'm very happy and very satisfied, and they're enthusiastic, and appear to be very knowledgeable. And that appears to be a workable alternative.

The only other thing that I would say is, and I've complained to AARP and whoever else I could think of, but this is a situation which—I consider myself to be a well-read individual, and I walked right into it, 3 years after I was 65 years old, not knowing about the issue, and it appears that—from the calls that I've made around, that the issue, or the problem, is well-known nationwide, it's just that very few people are talking about it, or addressing it. And that's all I have to say. Thank you.

Senator MURKOWSKI. Thank you, Mr. Westburg, I appreciate that. I think you're right. I think a lot of people get to that Medicare-eligible age, and realize that this is a problem that's been out there, but they just were simply not aware of it, and now they're in the middle of it.

I want to thank all of you for being with us this morning. We were scheduled to be out at noon, and it's noon straight up, so again, I want to thank you. There are some others who have indicated that they would like to submit testimony, and again, as I indicated this morning, we'll keep the record open here for several weeks for you to do that. I think we've received some written testimony already this morning, that will be included as part of the record.

Senator MURKOWSKI. But, I appreciate the perspective that so many of you have lent, whether it's from the consumer perspective, or whether from the provider perspective. And again, to those of you who are part of the residency program, part of the training program now, we welcome you, we thank you for your commitment to serve, and we wish you well. And we do, plead with you, to come back. We need you here.

And with that, we'll conclude the hearing.

[Additional material follows.]

ADDITIONAL MATERIAL

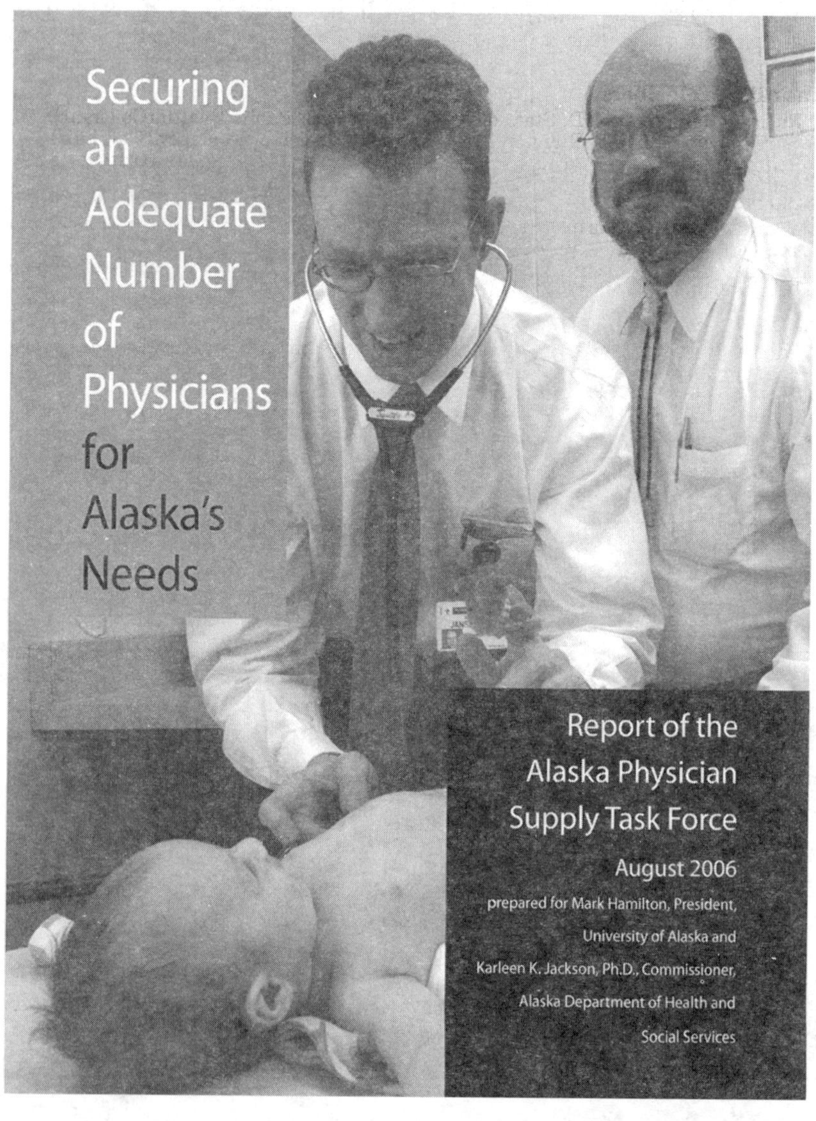

ACKNOWLEDGEMENTS

The Alaska Physician Supply Task Force wishes to thank the staff for their time, diligence, and expertise provided throughout this project. We also thank all those who contributed their knowledge and expertise in providing information and comments on our report.

Task Force Members

Richard Mandsager, MD, State of Alaska Director of Public Health (Co-Chair)
Harold Johnston, MD, Director, Alaska Family Medicine Residency (Co-Chair)
Rod Betit, President, Alaska State Hospital and Nursing Home Association
Jan Gehler, Ph.D., Interim Provost, University of Alaska Anchorage
David Head, MD, Medical Director, Norton Sound Health Corporation, and Chair, Alaska State Medical Board, representing Alaska Native Tribal Health Consortium
Jim Jordan, Executive Director, Alaska State Medical Association
Karen Perdue, Associate Vice President for Health Affairs, University of Alaska
Dennis Valenzeno, Ph.D., Director, Alaska WWAMI Biomedical Program

Staff

Patricia Can, Alice Rarig, Joyce Hughes, Stephanie Zidek-Chandler, and Jean Findley, from Health Planning and Systems Development Unit, Alaska Department of Health and Social Services, staffed the Task Force and coordinated production of the report.

Project Funding and Support

Funding to support the Alaska Physician Supply Task Force was provided by the University of Alaska Statewide, Office of the Associate Vice President for Health through Federal grants from the Health Resources and Services Administration, Office of Rural Health Policy, Special Projects (#D1ARH00052) and Centers for Disease Control (#H75/CCH024673-01). Additional funding for staff time was provided through the Department of Health and Social Services: Health Planning and Systems Development's Alaska Office of Rural Health (HRSA #H95RH00135), State Planning Grant (HRSA #PO9HSO5505), Primary Care Cooperative Agreement (HRSA #U68CSO0157), and Rural Hospital Flexibility Program (HRSA #H54RH00014).

The Task Force members acknowledge the resources that were provided by our own organizations. Our organizations have supported our time, travel and related in-kind resources for the project.

(Cover photo: Foreground, Andrew Janssen, M.D., a 2005 graduate of the Alaska Family Medicine Residency Program, examines 6-month-old Cooper Baines at the Providence Family Medicine Center in Anchorage, Alaska. Paul W. Davis, M.D., is shown in background. Photo by Greg Martin, 2005, courtesy of Providence Family Medicine Center.)

Securing an Adequate Number of Physicians for Alaska's Needs

REPORT OF THE ALASKA PHYSICIAN SUPPLY TASK FORCE

(Prepared for Mark Hamilton, President, University of Alaska and Karleen Jackson, Ph.D., Commissioner, Alaska Department of Health & Social Services August 2006)

TABLE OF CONTENTS

A. Emerging Trends and Issues Related to Physician Supply.
B. Forecasting the Need for Physicians in the Next Two Decades.
C. Reasons for Taking Action to Assure an Adequate Physician Supply.

A. Demographic Profile of Alaska through 2025.
B. Projected Demand and Supply of Physicians through 2025.

A. Medical School Opportunities for Alaskans.
B. Graduate Medical Education in Alaska—the Alaska Family Medicine Residency.
C. State, Federal and Tribal Efforts to Support Health Care Workforce Development.
D. Lessons from Other States and from National Studies.

A. Context and Process for Selection of Strategy Recommendations.
B. Goals and Strategy Recommendations
Goal 1. Increase the in-state production of physicians by increasing the number and viability of medical school and residency positions in Alaska and for Alaskans.
Goal 2. Increase the recruitment of physicians to Alaska by assessing needs and coordinating recruitment efforts.
Goal 3. Expand and support programs that prepare Alaskans for medical careers.
Goal 4. Improve retention of physicians by improving the practice environment in Alaska.

A. Data Details.
1. Matriculants in Medical Schools by State.
2. Specialty Distribution Comparison (2004) Alaska and US.
B. Strategies Preferences Scoresheet.
C. Physician Study Annotated Reference List.
D. Resource List.
E. Individual Contributors, Persons Consulted, Commenters, Reviewers, and Persons who Attended Task Force Meetings.
F. Acronym List.

LIST OF FIGURES

EXECUTIVE SUMMARY

The Alaska Physician Supply Task Force was commissioned in January 2006 by the President of the University of Alaska and the Commissioner of the Department of Health and Social Services to address two questions:

1. What is the current and future need for physicians in Alaska?

2. What strategies have been used and could be used in meeting the need for physicians in Alaska? Strategies of interest are:

- programs to attract and prepare students for health careers;
- medical school opportunities;
- graduate medical education; and
- recruitment and retention of physicians.

The Task Force has met regularly and drawn on a wide variety of sources of information, including public participation. The consensus of the Task Force is that this report represents the best answer possible to these questions, within the constraints of time and budget, and the inherent uncertainties of available data and predictions. The major conclusions and reasoning of the group are summarized here, and detailed in the body of the report.

Alaska has a shortage of physicians.[1] Although not at crisis levels, the shortage is affecting access to care throughout the State, and increasing cost to hospitals and health care organizations. Up to 16 percent of rural physician positions in Alaska were vacant in 2004. Patients with Medicare are having difficulty finding a primary care physician. Several important specialties are in serious shortage in Alaska.

The shortage is very likely to worsen over the next 20 years as the State's population increases and ages. Physician supply nationwide is entering a period of shortage, according to the best current predictions. Physicians in Alaska are aging and one-third may be retiring in the next 10–15 years. The new generation of physicians wants a more balanced life, meaning fewer hours on duty and more predictable schedules. These trends mean that more physicians will be required to serve the same population. Technology and scientific advances have increased the amount of medical care available, adding to the need for physicians, as the patients expect more care than previously.

As the national supply of physicians shrinks, recruitment will become more competitive. Alaska's traditional system of recruiting physicians from Federal assignment in the military and Indian Health Service is much less effective with changes in these systems. Although Alaska has two very successful programs to produce its own physicians, the Alaska WWAMI medical school program and the Alaska Family Medicine Residency, Alaska is far behind the other States in production capacity. These two programs, even if expanded, cannot meet the need.

The current trend in physician growth in Alaska is inadequate to keep up with basic population growth and to correct the current deficit. Unless changes are made in the systems used to increase physician numbers, the deficit will worsen, with significant consequences for access and quality of care for Alaskans, as well as increased cost for health care delivery systems.

The time frames to increase physician supply are long; it takes from 7 to 13 years from entry into medical school to entry into practice. The time it takes to develop new or expanded programs adds to this delay. It is important to act quickly to begin the programs that will yield more physicians in the next two decades. Delay will only add to the cost and worsen the deficit to recoup.

Responses to this problem involve preparing and attracting Alaskan youth so they can enter medical careers, improving recruitment of physicians to practice in Alaska, and retaining the physicians who currently practice here. The Task Force recommends specific strategies and action steps to achieve four goals related to assuring an adequate supply of physicians to meet Alaska's need.

Goals:

1. Increase the in-state production of physicians by increasing the number and viability of medical school and residency positions in Alaska and for Alaskans.

2. Increase the recruitment of physicians to Alaska by assessing needs and coordinating recruitment efforts.

3. Expand and support programs that prepare Alaskans for medical careers.

4. Increase retention of physicians by improving the practice environment in Alaska.

The following sections summarize the findings of the Alaska Physician Supply Task Force supporting these goals. The body of the report contains the full discus-

---

[1] Unless otherwise specified, "physician" in this report means medical doctor as well as doctor of osteopathy.

sion of the goals, strategy recommendations, and the rationale behind the recommendations.

Assessment of need. The Task Force estimates that Alaska has a shortage of 375 physicians, based on the conclusion that Alaska should have 110 percent of the current national average physician-to-population ratio. In order to correct the deficit and reach an adequate supply of physicians by 2025, Alaska needs to add a net of 59 physicians per year, starting immediately. Alaska currently gains 78 physicians per year but loses 40 physicians yearly for various reasons. In order to improve its doctor to population ratio, and assure having an adequate supply in 20 years, the current net gain of 38 physicians per year will need to increase to 59 per year, more than a 50 percent increase. If the loss each year is greater than the recent average of 40 per year, Alaska will need more than 90 physicians to enter practice in Alaska each year.

These conclusions are supported by the following findings.

Finding 1. The ratio of physicians to population in Alaska is below the national average at 2.05 MDs per 1,000 population vs. 2.38 MDs per 1000 population in the United States.

Finding 2. Alaska should have 10 percent more physicians per population than the national average because Alaska's rural nature, great distances and severe weather result in structural inefficiencies of the health care system. Alaskan physicians' administrative and supervisory responsibilities in addition to patient care contribute to the need for more physicians to provide patient care services.

Finding 3. Competition for physicians will intensify since the entire Nation is expected to experience a shortage of physicians, associated with the aging of the population and an inadequate production of physicians.

Finding 4. Retirement and practice reductions of aging physicians in Alaska and elsewhere, as well as changing preferences of physicians for more limited work hours, add to the need for more physicians.

Finding 5. Alaska has and should maintain a higher ratio of mid-level providers (advanced nurse practitioners and physician assistants) to physicians than the national average, in order to make it feasible to provide high quality and timely care to the population. Without these providers the need for physicians would be even higher.

Finding 6. Shortages are most apparent in internal medicine, medical subspecialties and psychiatry. It is important to evaluate the need for specialty types and distribution throughout Alaska, in order to plan for physician recruitment.

Over the next 20 years, nearly twice as many "physicians in practice" will be needed—about 1,100 more than the current 1,347 MDs in patient care—to meet expected demand as the State's elderly population triples and as medical practice patterns change. This projection assumes that doctors of osteopathy, advanced nurse practitioners and physician assistants will continue to increase proportionately over time.

Figure A. Gain in Alaskan Physicians: Static Doctor to Population Ratio vs. Desired Growth Scenario

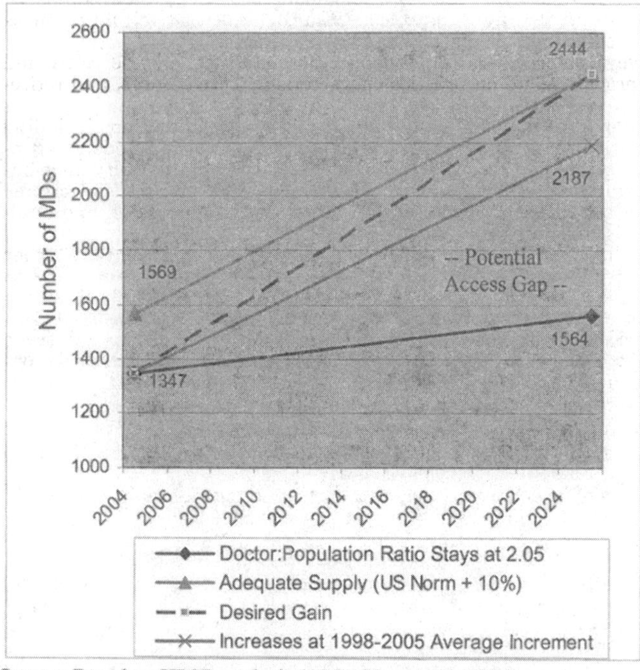

Source: Based on HPSD analysis (AMA Master File 2006)

Basis for strategies for meeting the need for physicians for Alaska's health care system. After investigating the supply and need for physicians and reaching Findings 1–6, the Task Force shifted its focus to investigating strategies for meeting the need. The Task Force drew on the knowledge of in-state professionals and educators, and of national experts, to identify lessons and information that form the basis for recommendations for action, as well as for further investigation and monitoring. The Task Force's selection of strategies is based on the following findings.

Finding 7. Alaska is one of six States without an independent in-state medical school. Alaska funds 10 state-supported "seats" at the regional WWAMI medical school, administratively centered at the University of Washington School of Medicine. This number (10 seats) represents fewer seats per capita than all but five of the 50 States.

Finding 8. Residency programs are one of the most effective ways to produce physicians for a State or community. Alaska has only one in-state residency, the AFMR, which places 70 percent of its graduates in Alaska. Maintaining and expanding residency opportunities will be critical in augmenting Alaska's physician numbers.

Finding 9. Over the last 10 years, an increasing number of Alaskan students have applied to medical schools; the average number of applicants has been 65. In 2005, 29 of 73 applicants were admitted into medical school. Ten per year attend WWAMI and the remainder attends medical schools without State support from Alaska. Since 1996, only WWAMI has had Alaska-supported seats. Prior to 1996, Alaska supported programs for medical and osteopathic students through the WICHE program and student loans.

Finding 10. Recruitment for physicians is facilitated by the availability of loan repayment programs such as the IHS and NHSC loan repayment programs. Service obligations related to student loans have historically accounted for some recruitment and should be explored.

Finding 11. There are several initiatives to increase interest in medical careers among Alaskans, including efforts by the tribal health care system, hospitals, the University of Alaska's newly funded Area Health Education Center (AHEC) and the UA Scholars Awards, school system initiatives for improvement of math and science programs, and programs that encourage students to go into health careers. Collectively, these initiatives generate qualified applicants to medical schools, but too few applicants matriculate to replenish Alaska's shortage, and there is inadequate diversity.

Finding 12. Medical practice environments in Alaska have positive and negative aspects that affect the recruitment and retention of physicians.

Finding 13. Surveys of providers (physicians and mid-levels) by the AMA and many States have provided data on practice characteristics, preferences, and retirement plans.

Finding 14. Workforce development activities exist in multiple locations including the tribally managed system, private sector, and various State and Federal agencies. However existing programs are not monitoring or analyzing specialty distribution or needs, changing roles of mid-level providers, or potential impact of electronic health records on all providers. Coordination of the efforts, and research and analysis of relevant trends, should inform policy.

In view of these findings, the relevant literature, and the experience of other States, the Task Force developed the following goals and strategies to respond to the physician shortage. The strategies are chosen because of their likely effectiveness, cost-to-benefit advantages, and achievability. Each strategy is discussed with respect to the time frame in which it will be effective, and the average expected cost to the State to produce each practicing physician, where such information is reasonably accessible. The listing below gives a brief identification of each goal and strategy. Full discussion of the strategies is included in the body of the report.

Goals and Strategies for Securing an Adequate Physician Supply for Alaska's Needs

Major goal	Strategy	Timeline for impact	Estimated cost
1. Increase the in-state production of physicians by increasing the number and viability of medical school and residency positions in Alaska and for Alaskans.	A. Increase the number of state-subsidized medical school positions (WWAMI) from 10 to 30 per year.	Medium	$250,000 per practicing physician.
	B. Ensure financial viability of the AFMR through State support including Medicaid support.	Short	$60,000 per practicing physician.
	C. Increase the number of residency positions in Alaska, both in family medicine and appropriate additional specialties.	Short	$100,000 per year plus $30,000 for planning in year 1 & 2.
	D. Assist Alaskan students to attend medical school by: (i) reactivating and funding the use of the WICHE Professional Student Exchange Program with a service obligation attached, and (ii) evaluating the possibility of seats for Alaskans in the planned osteopathic school at the Pacific Northwest University of the Health Science.	Medium	(i) $550,000 per practicing physician for WICHE; (ii) cost unknown at time of PSTF report.
	E. Investigate mechanisms for increasing Alaska-based experiences and education for WWAMI Students.	Medium	Unknown at time of PSTF Report.
	F. Maximize Medicare payments to teaching hospitals in Alaska.	Short	Zero cost to the State.
	G. Empanel a group to assess medical education in Alaska, including the viability of establishing an Alaska-based medical school.	Long	Undetermined at time of PSTF Report.
2. Increase the recruitment of physicians to Alaska by assessing needs and coordinating recruitment efforts.	A. Create a Medical Provider Workforce Assessment Office to monitor physician supply and facilitate physician recruitment efforts.	Short	$250,000 per year.
	B. Research and test a physician relocation incentive payment program.	Short	$65,000 per physician.

Goals and Strategies for Securing an Adequate Physician Supply for Alaska's Needs—Continued

Major goal	Strategy	Timeline for impact	Estimated cost
	C. Expand loan repayment assistance programs and funding for physicians practicing in Alaska.	Short	Undetermined—need to consult with other States.
3. Expand and support programs that prepare Alaskans for medical careers.	A. Expand and coordinate programs that prepare Alaskans for careers in medicine.	Medium	Up to $1,000,000 per year.
4. Increase retention of physicians by improving the practice environment in Alaska.	A. Develop a physician practice environment index for Alaska.	Short	$100,000 to develop index; $20,000 annually to update.
	B. Develop tools that promote community-based approaches to physician recruitment and retention.	Short	$50,000 per year.
	C. Support Federal tax credit legislation Initiative for physicians that meet frontier practice requirements.	Short	Zero cost to the State.

Adoption of these strategies will depend on further analysis of resources and a balancing of effectiveness and achievability. Strategies to recruit and retain physicians promise the earliest positive results, but probably have a relatively low benefit ceiling, in that the maximum number of physicians achievable by those strategies will soon be reached. The strategies likely to produce significant numbers of doctors over time are those designed to train physicians in Alaska, i.e. medical school and residency programs, but the time to realize the benefit in most cases is longer.

Implementation strategy—next steps for key policymakers. The shortage of physicians and other health care providers creates one of Alaska's most challenging public health and higher education issues. To ensure the work of the Task Force is carried forward, it is recommended that the President and Commissioner establish permanent structures to implement these recommendations. One component of this action would be creation of a Medical Provider Workforce Assessment Office (Strategy 2A).

SECTION I. OVERVIEW: THE PHYSICIAN SUPPLY TASK FORCE APPROACH

In December 2005, University of Alaska President Mark Hamilton and Alaska Department of Health and Social Services Commissioner Karleen Jackson appointed the Alaska Physician Supply Task Force to answer two primary questions.

1. What is the current and future need for physicians in Alaska?

2. What strategies have been used and could be used in meeting the need for physicians in Alaska? Strategies of interest are:

- programs to attract and prepare students for health careers;
- medical school opportunities;
- graduate medical education; and
- recruitment and retention of physicians.

The Task Force as a group of experts, was charged by President Hamilton and Commissioner Jackson to recommend the most appropriate and effective response to a persistent physician supply shortage within Alaska, spiraling costs of recruitment, effects on Alaska of projected national shortfalls, and the need to develop a workable plan to meet physician workforce needs throughout the State from now through 2025.

The Physician Supply Task Force worked through two phases:

- Phase I (December 2005—March 2006); and
- Phase II (February 2006—August 2006).

During Phase I the Task Force identified and analyzed the data regarding medical provider counts for the State and compared it to data from other States and nationwide. This phase assisted in evaluating the scope of the problem. The Task Force also considered the expertise of its members, and the knowledge of other advisors and consultants from Alaska regarding State programs for encouraging students to enter health careers, for subsidizing or contributing to training programs, and for supporting students through scholarships and loans.

In Phase II the Task Force chose to focus on developing short, medium and long term recommendations to meet physician supply requirements in Alaska through 2025. They also considered the impact of their recommendations on training, recruitment and retention of physicians. The Task Force prioritized and grouped strategies based on reports from other States, Alaska's experience, and expected feasibility and effectiveness in the current environment.

Task Force members chose to operate under a consensus model related to findings and strategies. During their work, the Task Force members used scoring methodologies, expert testimony, and staff consultation to reach their findings and recommendations.

Task Force members and invited guests shared their expertise regarding training of physicians. Presentations included those from WWAMI (Washington, Wyoming, Alaska, Montana and Idaho) regional medical school based within the University of Washington School of Medicine, and the AFMR in Anchorage.

Staff contacted experts from the Center for Health Workforce Studies at the University of Washington, the North Carolina Rural Health Research Program and Program on Health Policy Analysis at the University of North Carolina at Chapel Hill, the Utah Medical Education Council, and other State and national programs. Reports of the several Centers for Health Workforce Studies, U.S. Bureau of Labor Statistics, Health Resources and Services Administration, and other States that have addressed physician workforce issues were studied. A review of the literature focused on assessing and forecasting physician supply and demand at State and national levels, and on strategies being used to increase physician supply. Current status of recruitment and retention efforts and programs such as student loan programs and loan forgiveness options that have been used in Alaska and elsewhere were reviewed.

The Task Force met monthly from December 2005 to August 2006. Public comment was encouraged throughout the process. Meeting announcements were publicly posted and time was set aside at each meeting for public comment. In addition to monthly meetings, a longer meeting was held March 27, 2006 to discuss, enhance and prioritize recommnendations. This meeting included a broad group including stakeholders, members of the public, and Task Force and project staff. The draft report was distributed for review and comment to over ninety individuals who have expertise and interest in this issue.

The next three sections of the report describe current information from diverse sources in Alaska about trends and issues related to physician supply and recruitment, distribution, and factors in Alaska that may need to be considered in forecasting need, followed by more detailed information about the data that can be used to forecast supply. This material provides the basis for the "findings" relating to the first question asked of the Task Force: "What is the current and future need for physicians in Alaska?" Section V provides the information gathered to answer the second question: "What strategies have been used and could be used in meeting the need for physicians in Alaska?" Section VI contains detailed discussions of the goals and strategies proposed by the Task Force. Section VII includes a listing of areas that warrant further consideration, in that they were discussed by the Task Force but not researched or thoroughly documented in this report.

SECTION II. BACKGROUND: STATE AND NATIONAL TRENDS IN UNDERSTANDING
PHYSICIAN SUPPLY AND DEMAND

Alaska's health care organizations are facing major difficulties and great expense in recruiting and retaining physicians. Both private and public health care agencies have pointed out to State policymakers and the University of Alaska that they are spending increasing time and money seeking doctors to staff their services. A looming national shortage is already affecting Alaska's service delivery. Indeed, a review of the literature finds that the United States is experiencing a shortage of physicians which is predicted to rise due to the needs of an aging population, increases in physician retirement, restricted production of new physicians nationally, insufficient GME training capacity, and changes in practice patterns. By 2020, a deficit of 96,000 to 200,000 doctors is anticipated nationwide (Cooper, 2004).

History of national physician shortage. The current shortage can be traced back to a response to a series of influential reports published between 1981 and the mid 1990s, which inaccurately predicted that the Nation would experience a large surplus of physicians by 2000. The reports were written by national advisory groups, including the Graduate Medical Education National Advisory Committee (GMENAC) and the Council on Graduate Medical Education (COGME), that were tasked with making policy recommendations regarding the adequacy of the supply and distribution of physicians (Cooper, 2004).[2] Their information was driven by an opinion that health maintenance organizations (HMOs) would decrease physician demand by promoting preventive care and reducing tests and procedures.

Subsequent to these reports, allopathic medical schools around the country voluntarily capped the production of new physicians. However, residency programs and osteopathic medical schools did not heed the reports' warnings and continued to increase the number of physicians in the residency programs and osteopathic schools. Between 1980 and 1990, the number of residents training in the U.S. increased by nearly 50 percent from 62,000 to 92,000 residents (Salsberg and Forte, 2002).

As concerns about physician oversupply escalated, COGME recommended in 1996 that the number of physicians entering residency programs be reduced from 140 percent to 110 percent of the baseline (the number of medical school graduates in 1993) and that the percentage of specialists to generalists be evenly split, 50/50. Finally, in 1997, Congress placed a cap on the number of available residency slots that would be supported by the Medicare program. This significant economic disincentive effectively capped GME in the United States.

It was not long, however, before the wisdom of these recommendations and subsequent restrictive policies was questioned. Physician oversupply did not occur. Instead, reports of shortages for both general practitioners and specialists surfaced (Schubert et al., 2003; Miller et al., 2001). It appeared that a significant shortage rather than oversupply was looming on the horizon. As a result, COGME reviewed physician workforce projections again, predicted that physician demand would significantly outpace supply, and recommended that medical schools expand the number of graduates by 3,000 per year by 2015. In 2005, the executive council of the Association of American Medical Colleges (AAMC) called for a 15 percent increase in medical school enrollment, and in June, 2006, the AAMC called for a 30 percent increase in medical school slots by 2020 in order to meet future physician needs (AAMC, 2006).

Economic impact of physician supply. The supply of physicians impacts State economies in many ways. It is an economic driver and affects a State's ability to draw businesses as well as skilled, competitive employees. Businesses and potential staff are more likely to locate in communities that assure the availability of quality medical care services. Dollars spent on health care are recycled in the economy to the extent that labor, supplies and services are acquired locally. In 2004, personal health care expenditures represented 13.4 percent of the gross national product. It represented 12.3 percent (1.6 billion dollars) of Alaska's gross State product. (*www.cms.hhs.gov/NationalHealthExpendData/downloads/ nhestatesummary2004.pdf*)

In Alaska, business concern about adequacy of health services in the State has been expressed by the Commonwealth North study of primary care and the subsequent initiatives in 2005–2006 of the Alaska Health Care Roundtable to examine costs of health care and health insurance, and availability of options for employers and employees (Commonwealth North, 2005). The University of Alaska, Institute for Social and Economic Research recently produced an analysis of costs of health care in Alaska (UA ISER, 2006). The Alaska State Medical Association (ASMA), the Alaska State Hospital and Nursing Home Association (ASHNA), the University of Alaska, and the State's largest health care organizations (Providence Health Systems and the Alaska Native Tribal Health Consortium (ANTHC)) have all focused on the looming shortage and have begun to take steps to improve practice environments.

SECTION III. THE ALASKA STORY: HISTORICAL AND CURRENT INFORMATION ON
PHYSICIAN SUPPLY

A. Emerging Trends and Issues Related to Physician Supply

In 2004, Alaska's physician-to-population ratio ranked 17th lowest in the Nation—i.e., in the lower third of all States.[3][4] About 1,350 allopathic physicians (MDs)

---

[2] Richard Cooper MD has written extensively on the evolution and effect of these positions and reports. See Annals of Intern Med 141, 2004, p. 705.

[3] Allopathic medicine is conventional medicine. The term was coined in 1842 by C.F.S. Hahnemann to designate the usual practice of medicine as opposed to homeopathy. Doctors of osteopathy have completed a course of study equivalent to that of an MD and are licensed to practice medicine. They may prescribe medication and perform surgery, and they often use manipulation techniques similar to chiropractics or physical therapy.

[4] Chen et al., 2005 show Alaska in the middle of the range of States using the 2005 AMA master file, selecting "clinically active" physicians, but using a slightly lower population estimate than that used in this report. Kaiser Family Foundation "statehealthfacts.org" and the U.S. Statistical Abstract show rankings using counts of "non-Federal physicians" only. Since

work in patient care and about 100 osteopathic physicians (DOs) are in practice in Alaska. Alaska has 205 physicians (MDs and DOs) providing patient care per 100,000 population, compared with 238 for the United States (AMA, 2006).

A recent survey of "vacant" slots for Alaska physicians indicated a 16 percent vacancy rate outside of Anchorage. Although doctors of osteopathy, advanced nurse practitioners and physician assistants are available in Alaska to provide medical care, the current deficit in allopathic physicians is being felt by the profession and by health care organizations as they seek to staff their services. The current "shortage" using the national physician to population ratio as the norm can be defined as equal to 218 fewer physicians currently in patient care in Alaska than if the U.S. ratio applied.

Figure 1. A First Look at Physician Count in Alaska

Measure	MD Count (Alaska)	MDs Per 1000 Population
2004 actual physicians in patient care (per AMA Master File)	1,347	2.05
2004 "expected" at national average	1,565	2.38
"Deficit" from national norm	218	---
Percent "deficit"	14 percent	---
Outside Anchorage Vacancy Rate (AFMR survey 2004)	16 percent	---

Alaska's specialists are located mainly in the largest urban centers. Anchorage, which serves as the specialty center for the State as a whole, has approximately 464 specialists and 323 "primary care" physicians (family practitioners, internists, pediatricians and obstetrician-gynecologists).[5] Anecdotal information suggests that Anchorage lacks sufficient primary care physicians, especially internists, to meet the population's needs. The Task Force identified this as one area needing further study.

Rural areas are served by primary care physicians who are headquartered mostly in regional centers. In rural census areas and boroughs there are fewer physicians per population than in the urban areas. Telehealth development in Alaska has improved the ability of physicians in regional centers to supervise and consult with mid-level providers in sub-regional and village clinics, and with community health aides and practitioners in the Alaska tribal health care system. Similarly, the telehealth options have enabled primary care physicians in rural areas to consult with specialists in Anchorage and in some cases out-of-state experts. Within both the tribal system and the private sector, there are still itinerant specialists (both in-state and out-of-state residents) who visit rural communities or regional centers to hold specialty clinics or see selected patients. The regionalized structure provides for a level of access to care that could not be supported economically by individual communities.

Small communities typically have a difficult time supporting physician services, in Alaska as well as elsewhere. Communities may be "too small, too poor, or too disadvantaged in geographic competition to support sufficient viable physician practices," and may not have the "economic wherewithal to support more physician practices even though physician to population ratios may indicate they are needed" (Wright et al., 2001). Seasonal fluctuations related to tourism, fishing season, and weather-dependent construction are often an additional challenge to small Alaskan communities. Staffing levels which may be appropriate on average through a year may be inadequate for peak periods, which can also "burn out" an isolated, solo provider. National trends are away from solo practices. Alaska is also experiencing trends toward hospital hires of physicians, reliance on emergency medicine specialists to staff emergency rooms, and clinics having a combination of physician and mid-level (advanced nurse practitioner and physician assistants) staffing.

Distribution of Alaska physicians. The Task Force has recognized that there are inherent inefficiencies related to the vast distances that must be covered by patients and providers, uncertainties of weather and transportation options, and the inherent challenges of living and working in remote and geographically isolated conditions. These factors were considered in Task Force deliberations about targets for

---

these use population estimates that include the military and Alaska Native and American Indian populations who are served by the excluded physicians, the resulting rankings placing Alaska lower than 17th. These differences show the importance of understanding the definitions of the inputs and assumptions made in any presentation of similar data.

[5] DHSS Health Planning and Systems Development analysis of occupational licensing and ASMA data (merged).

physician supply. Figure 2 shows the distribution of physicians and population for areas with five or more physicians.

Figure 2. Distribution of Alaska Physicians by City and Percent in Primary Care

City/Area of Physicians in Alaska	Total Physicians	State's Physicians in the City (percent)	Physicians in the City who are in Primary Care (percent)	Alaska Population in the City/Area (percent)
Anchorage Total	787	60	41	42
Fairbanks Total	151	11	51	13
Wasilla, Palmer, Willow	83	6	49	11
Juneau/Auke Bay	70	5	46	5
Soldotna & Kenai	46	3	52	7
Sitka	31	2	68	1
Ketchikan	27	2	56	2
Kodiak	23	2	74	2
Homer	18	1	44	1
Bethel	15	1	100	4
Dillingham	8	1	100	1
Nome	8	1	88	1
Kotzebue	6	0	100	1
Seward	6	0	83	1
Barrow	5	0	80	1
Balance of State	32	2		7
Total with known spec'ty	1,316	100		

Note: Primary Care physicians include family practitioners, internists, pediatricians and obstetrician-gynecologists.

Source: Merged ASMA Directory listing and Alaska Occupational Licensing database (AKDHSS HPSD 2006).

It should be noted that Anchorage has a higher percent of the State's physicians for their population because it is Alaska's largest city and is a specialty referral center. Many patients come to Anchorage from other parts of the State for medical care. Fairbanks, Juneau, Sitka, Kenai/Soldotna and Ketchikan each have several specialties represented among the physicians.

Fluctuations in physician supply. The Task Force has examined the data on licensing of new physicians in the State and loss of resident physicians, measured by expiration of licenses or moves out of state. Losses are attributable to retirement, migration, and mortality. Detailed findings are described below in analysis of trends.

The ASMA Directory showed a drop in listed physicians in 2004, prompting discussion and concern. (See Figure 3.) The decline was explained by a sudden drop in the listed members of the military services, related to the base closings and deployments to Iraq.

**Figure 3. Change from Prior Year in Total Physicians, by Practice Type
Alaska 1997-2005**

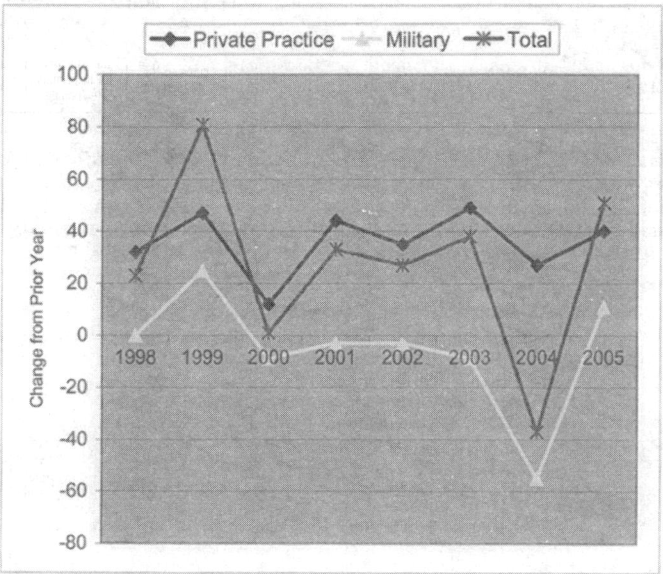

Source: ASMA Directories 1997-2005

A critical finding of the Task Force has been that since 1998 new MD licenses have averaged 78 per year, and on average 40 licenses have expired each year.[6]

Physician recruitment in Alaska appears to have declined since a high point in 2002 (there were 108 new MD licenses for physicians with Alaskan addresses in 2002 and only 73 in 2005). Licenses of new DOs have been increasing (from six in 1998 to nine in 2005), and numbers of advanced nurse practitioners and physician assistants being licensed annually have increased as well (see Figure 4).

Figure 4. New Licensees Annually 1996–2005 by Type

(Active Licenses, Alaska Addresses, in practice in January 2006)

	MD	DO	NP	PA
1996	68	1	18	15
1997	65	7	26	14
1998	86	6	28	19
1999	92	8	18	9
2000	67	5	32	13
2001	71	4	25	11
2002	108	8	25	22
2003	90	7	30	12
2004	61	11	32	39
2005	73	9	30	29

Note: From comparative data for 1998 it is evident that some of the earlier licensees have left Alaska or left practice. To do a precise and complete analysis would require analysis of the "comments" files kept by Occupational Licensing, which was not feasible during this project.

Source: Alaska Division of Occupational Licensure

---

[6] The number of both new and expired licenses has varied from year to year (see Figure 4), with new licensees ranging from a high of 108 in 2002 to 61 in 2004. The timing of losses to the State's physician supply is more difficult to pinpoint than entry since out-movers or retirees may not report changes in address or activity to the Alaska State Medical Board immediately. When they do report, the information is entered as "comments" with the status change noted, but the details about the date and specific reasons for change would need to be analyzed through a study of the Board's detailed file "comment" entries. These are not part of the publicly available electronic files.

If the number of Alaska physicians retiring increases, or out-migration or "lapsing" of licenses increases, Alaska could lose more physicians than it gains, adding to the burden of boosting the current supply. The Status of Recruitment Resources and Strategies report indicated rapidly escalating costs of recruitment for rural physicians, and increased dependence on *locum tenens* physicians to handle patient care (DHSS/ACRH, 2006).

Two trends could intensify the need for new physician recruits in Alaska. One trend is that the physician workforce is aging, so the rate of retirement is likely to increase, thus increasing the loss of physicians. The second trend is the growing national shortage, which is already making recruitment to Alaska more difficult.

B. Forecasting the Need for Physicians in the next Two Decades

According to the Task Force projections of need (elaborated in Section IV below), at this time Alaska needs a net gain of about 59 new physicians each year to offset the number of physicians who leave or retire. Annual losses are currently 40 per year, but are expected to increase as a higher proportion of physicians age and retire. One "linear" scenario for replacing physicians as they leave practice, and building the total supply, is illustrated in Figure 5. A net gain of 59 physicians per year would be a 50 percent increase over the recent average net gain of 38 per year. This increment could be accomplished by increasing the number of new licensees to average between 100 and 105 per year.

Figure 5. A Linear Growth Scenario for Physician Supply

Year	Projected Physicians in Practice			Needed Annual Increment	Estimated Loss due to Migration/ Retirement	Recruitment Needed to Achieve Needed Increment
	MDs in Practice	DOsActive	Total			
2004	1,347	109	1,456	59	40	99
2005	1,399	115	1,515	59	40	99
2006	1,451	122	1,573	59	41	100
2007	1,504	128	1,632	59	41	100
2008	1,556	135	1,690	59	42	101
2009	1,608	141	1,749	59	42	101
2010	1,660	147	1,808	59	43	102
2011	1,712	154	1,866	59	43	102
2012	1,765	160	1,925	59	44	103
2013	1,817	167	1,983	59	44	103
2014	1,869	173	2,042	59	45	104
2015	1,921	179	2,101	59	45	104
2016	1,973	186	2,159	59	46	105
2017	2,026	192	2,218	59	46	105
2018	2,078	199	2,276	59	47	106
2019	2,130	205	2,335	59	47	106
2020	2,182	211	2,394	59	48	107
2021	2,234	218	2,452	59	48	107
2022	2,287	224	2,511	59	49	108
2023	2,339	231	2,569	59	49	108
2024	2,391	237	2,628	59	50	109
2025	2,444	244	2,688	59	50	109

More physicians are needed for the following reasons: to correct the current deficit, to keep up with population growth, to address increased demand and need associated with aging of the population, and to compensate for changing practice patterns that are resulting in less time available for patient care on the part of the physicians in practice. Nationally the practice pattern changes are adding to the need for higher numbers of physicians in practice per 1,000 population, even where the number of "full time equivalents" might be relatively stable (HRSA, 2005; Bureau of Labor Statistics, 2006). Such practice patterns include:

• physician preferences for salaried positions with fewer hours in patient care and "on call";

• reduced hours for older physicians (nationally it has been noted that older physicians reduce their average hours, whether by shortening office hours, reducing patient rosters, bringing on partners, or taking more vacations);

• more "job sharing" by physicians;

- longer office visits and/or more time devoted to group sessions with patients as part of efforts to improve clinical prevention counseling;
- more time devoted to consults and supervision and training of other health workers; and
- other changes that may improve productivity of the system as a whole but not increase patient care productivity of the physician workforce, itself.

Alaska's rural physicians face additional challenges. Approximately 75 percent of Alaskan communities are not connected by road to another community with a hospital. Geography and climate together limit transportation options for providers and patients. Health care services for the rural population have evolved with a regional model where physicians and hospitals are located mostly in regional centers. A number of mid-level providers work in sub-regional centers, generally the largest "villages" in their areas, or serve villages on an itinerant basis from the regional or sub-regional clinics. In most villages populated by Alaska Natives, a community health aide or practitioner serves immediate behavioral and physical health needs, referring patients to higher level providers or using telehealth consults as needed.

These arrangements result in physicians serving more of their time in a consultative and oversight role than in typical settings in the Nation. In addition to such differences in practice responsibilities, rural physicians (almost all family practitioners rather than specialists) have to handle the entire spectrum of needs. They must often decide on and arrange for referrals to specialists located in distant cities. The poverty and hazardous occupations of Alaska's remote areas also contribute to high levels of need. These circumstances must be considered in determining a reasonable expectation for physician to population ratios.

C. Reasons for Taking Action to Assure an Adequate Physician Supply

In Alaska as well as throughout the Nation, there are mounting concerns about patients facing dangerously long wait times even for primary care physicians. Wait times for specialty care doctors are even longer and reflect the emerging strain. A system unable to provide timely medical care is certain to have a deleterious impact on health outcomes and further erode long-term population health goals.

> *Many patients, especially elderly patients on Medicare, are having difficulty finding a primary care physician. Most Internal Medicine physicians cannot afford to take on new Medicare patients because Medicare payment rates are so low. In addition, salaries of sub-specialists are much higher and discourage physicians from going into Internal Medicine. Generalists are being starved out.*
> —RICHARD NEUBAUER, MD, INTERNAL MEDICINE, ANCHORAGE, AMERICAN COLLEGE OF PHYSICIANS, BOARD OF REGENTS.

Increasing access to comprehensive high quality health care services is a key goal of the Healthy Alaskans 2010 plan. Reaching that goal depends upon having an adequate supply of doctors practicing in Alaska, having an appropriate distribution of physicians geographically to support the systems in place including mid-level providers and community health aides and practitioners in remote communities, and having an appropriate distribution of specialists to provide the continuum of services needed. Specific shortages of internists, psychiatrists (for adults and children), and certain medical sub-specialties have been reported to the Task Force. Comparisons of specialists per 1,000 population confirmed the large differences in availability of these providers in Alaska compared with the United States as a whole.

Key factors that will exacerbate the Alaska deficit include:

- aging of the population. Alaska's population over age 65 is expected to nearly triple by 2025 (Williams, 2005);
- aging physician workforce;
- increased competition among States to recruit from a limited supply of physicians;
- practice changes (such as preferences for fixed hours and limited number of hours) that further increase the number of physicians needed to meet adequately the health care needs of the State's population; and
- patients' increasing expectations for diagnosis and treatment.

Availability of health services in an area affects demographics of communities and of Alaska as a whole. Historically, the percentage of Alaskan residents over age 65 has been lower than in most States (6 percent in Alaska in 2005 compared with 12 percent nationwide). Although much of this difference has been related to high mortality rates of Alaska Natives and the in-migration of adults in the 1980–1985 oil boom who are just now reaching retirement age, another explanation has been that many older Alaskans have moved either to the cities or out-of-state because they were unable to have their health care needs met in their home communities. Improved availability of physicians including internists and specialists in the diseases that affect older people is likely to affect the rate of out-migration of senior citizens.

National workforce projections indicate that the shortage of physicians is escalating, although the gap could be held close to constant if medical schools and residencies expand.[7] Since the lead-time for preparing a college graduate to practice medicine is 7 years, policymakers need to consider promptly any indication of an emerging shortage of physicians.

SECTION IV. FINDINGS AND METHODS FOR FORECASTING SUPPLY AND DEMAND TO 2025 IN ALASKA

A. Demographic Profile of Alaska Through 2025

Alaska's 664,000 population in 2005 included about 37,000 new residents since 2000, or a 6 percent increase in 5 years. The most recent population projections for Alaska indicate an increase to about 788,000 by 2025—another 124,000 people— about 1 percent (7,000) increase per year. Population projections are based on patterns of birth, death and migration that are evident or expected based on recent trends and on anticipated economic developments known at the time the projections are made. (To account for some of the uncertainty, Alaska's demographer provides a "low" and "high" projection series as well. For 2020 the "low" projection is 712,000, the "high" is 823,000.) In addition to its resident population, Alaska hosts over a million tourist visitors a year, and hundreds of thousands of people who come to the State or its waters to work in fishing and fish processing, tourism, extractive industries, and other activities. Alaska also has seasonal residents who are not included in census counts of the resident population.

One quarter of the resident population lives in approximately 321 places that have fewer than 2,500 people. Most of these communities are geographically isolated from not only each other but also from the "urban" hub communities that have health care facilities including staff at the mid-level or physician level. The geography and demographic distributions of small populations of these communities as well as some communities on the "road system," are challenges that underlie the effort to provide access to health care in an extreme frontier State with 1.1 persons per square mile in 353 communities.

---

[7] The shortage hypothesis is not universally accepted. Starfield, Salsberg, Blumenthal, Elison and others have pointed out that health status is not directly correlated with physician to population ratios (many countries with lower ratios have better health status than the United States, for example) but in some instances a higher ratio of primary care to specialists is associated with better health status; they point to systems changes including broader roles for ANPs and PAs, electronic health records, more effective health promotion and clinical prevention approaches, holding down the need for higher physician to population ratios even if physicians practice shorter hours and retire earlier and at higher rates.

Figure 6. Population Projection for Alaskans Over Age 65

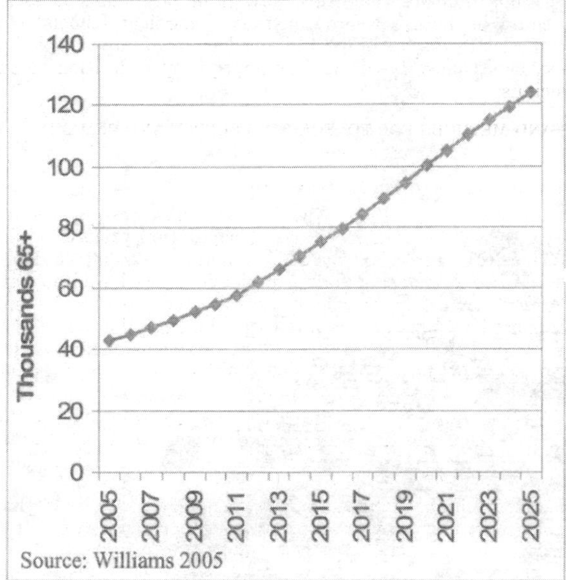

Assuming that age-specific migration and mortality patterns will remain similar to the current (2000–2005) patterns, it is projected that the population aged 65 and older will nearly triple by 2025, from about 43,000 people in 2005 to about 124,000 in 2025. The State Demographer has noted: "Given the lag time necessary to train occupations such as nurses, already in short supply, and to expand home care and assisted living, major efforts to meet what is already becoming a crisis in the State cannot begin too soon. The impact of the rapidly increasing numbers of older residents may be greater than elsewhere, because Alaska, with its historically younger population and relatively small number of elders, has fewer existing resources to serve the elderly" (Williams, 2005). Aged dependency (currently 10 elders per 100 Alaskans of working age) is expected to nearly triple by 2025, while child dependency will increase from the current level of 46 to about 49 children per 100 working age adults.

Figure 7. Alaska Population Projection by Age and Male/Female, 2024

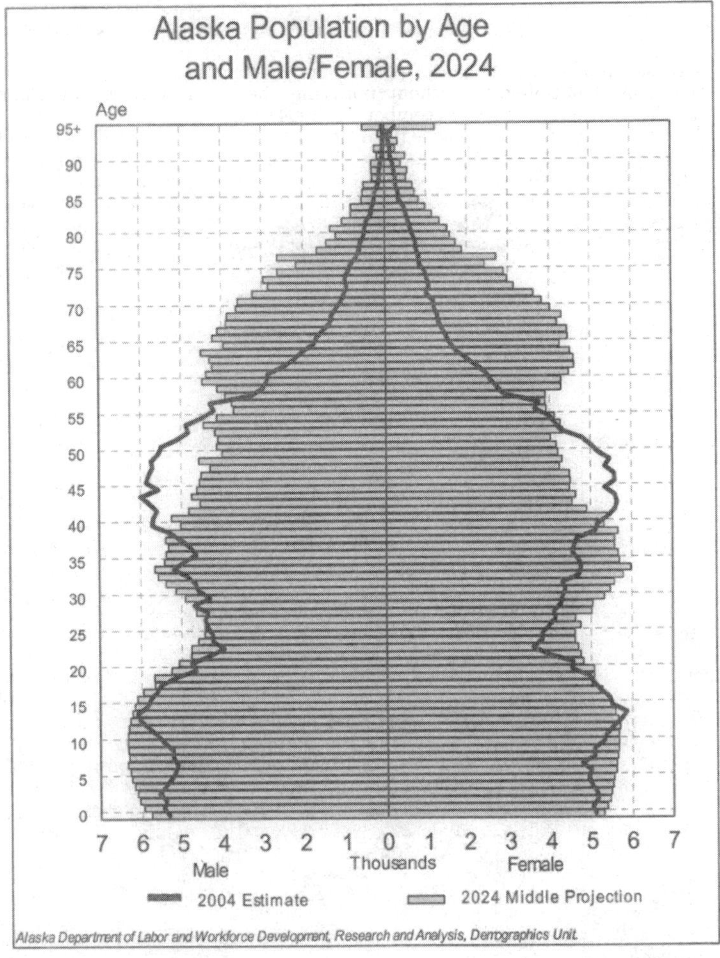

While the age distribution of the population changes in the next two decades, the health risks associated with both age and occupation may change. Alaska's economy relies considerably on oil extraction, fisheries, fish processing, tourism and mining, which include seasonally variable work and many occupations with high risk of injury.

A trend to more service sector jobs may reduce the rate of occupational injuries and death, but may also be associated with limited health insurance benefits. A continuing trend toward the service sector jobs may contribute to a drop in average median household income, and increases in the percentage uninsured. There may be a higher demand for health care if better health insurance coverage is available in the future, for all age groups. Risks for chronic disease have been increasing generally, so the needs for clinical preventive work as well as diagnosis, treatment and therapeutic services are likely to grow considerably.

B. Projected Demand and Supply of Physicians Through 2025

Current physician mid-level counts. This report describes, references and summarizes three independent sources of data about physicians in Alaska, including the State of Alaska Occupational Licensing database, ASMA directory listing (includes association members and non-members), and the American Medical Association (AMA) Master File. Strengths and limitations of each source are noted.

According to the State of Alaska Division of Occupational Licensing, 1,392 allopathic physicians (MDs), and 109 doctors of osteopathy (DOs) have Alaska addresses and "AA" (active) status, for a total of 1,501 physicians, or 2.26 physicians per thousand residents. However, the true supply of Alaskan physicians is actually smaller, as these figures include those not actively providing patient care, as well as those who moved out-of-state without notifying the Medical Licensing Board since the last license renewal date (December 31, 2004).[8]

A second source of data is the ASMA directory, which lists a total of 1,414 MDs and DOs (as of January 2006), of whom 1,221 are "active." This database appears to slightly underestimate the actual supply of Alaskan physicians, despite the fact that it includes both members and non-members of the Association. A comparison of the ASMA database and the State of Alaska Occupational Licensing database indicates that the ASMA list excludes some military physicians as well as a number of physicians working in the Alaska tribal health care system who are licensed in the State.

Both of the ASMA and State of Alaska Occupational Licensing databases specify whether a physician is "active" (ASMA) or "AA" (Occupational Licensing). However, there is no standard definition for active status in either database. Therefore, the databases may include physicians practicing less than 20 hours a week, or active in non-patient care work such as administration, teaching or research.

A third independent source is the AMA Master File of Allopathic Physicians (MDs), which counted 1,580 physicians in Alaska in 2004, of whom 1,347 are reported to be actively engaged in patient care (20 hours a week or more). This database is the only known source with standardized definitions uniformly applied to physicians throughout the United States. As such, the Physician Supply Task Force uses the physician supply data from this database for purposes of working toward an "Alaska Standard" physician-to-population ratio. The AMA Master File tracks physicians from medical school onward. It counts primary location and primary specialty. Since the AMA also obtains information about practice activity that permits distinguishing providers "active in patient care" for 20 hours a week or more, it provides a more accurate estimate of physicians providing care to the population than the other available sources. The Task Force uses the data based on the 2004 AMA survey for comparisons of "active allopathic physicians in patient care" with other States and with the Nation as a whole. Separate data from Occupational Licensing and from the professional associations is provided about doctors of osteopathy and mid-level providers.

Retirement status is reported in all three databases. In Alaska, a physician may let a license "lapse" by not renewing, for example when starting retirement, but may within 2 years of the license expiration date request reinstatement without penalty. After a 2-year lapse, re-licensure must begin as if the individual had never been licensed in Alaska before.

The Task Force recognizes that of the 109 DOs with Alaska addresses, 77 percent (84) work in primary care (Occupational Licensing database). This is a substantially higher percentage than the 60 percent reported nationally.[9] Ninety-two (92) active DOs are listed by ASMA. Among the DOs active in Alaska as of early 2006, about five had come into the State each year during the 1990s. That number increased to seven per year for licenses awarded in 2000–2005, or one new DO license for every 11 MD licenses.

Each of the available databases thus provides useful information. Since detailed analysis of the AMA Master File would require a costly purchase, it has not been feasible to use that source for regional or other detailed analysis. It is possible to compare the specialty distributions between the AMA and ASMA databases, and to check for consistency between the age distributions for physicians included in the licensing database as "active" and those in the AMA Master File. The Task Force has been able to analyze the occupational licensing database merged with the ASMA listing of members and non-members known to be practicing in Alaska, as of January 2006. The occupational licensing database has birth date of provider, while the

---

[8] Nearly 1,000 additional physicians (MD and DO) have active licenses to practice in Alaska but do not have Alaska addresses. These include physicians who work periodically as *locum tenens* practitioners, some who visit the State to provide specialty services on an itinerant basis, physicians licensed in Alaska in order to provide telemedicine consults for Alaska patients, others who may not visit on any regular basis, some who have left the State but maintain their license, and some who have obtained a license but decided not to practice in the State.

[9] Memo to Alaska Task Force, March 27, 2006 from Byron Perkins, DO, President, AKOMA.

ASMA database has activity type and declared primary specialty. It should be noted that the "counts" might differ slightly (see Figure 8).

Figure 8. Active Physicians by Degree Type

Physician Degree Type	Private Practice, Military, Public Health (Excludes retirees, residents, and those who report State and Federal Number rather than PH)	Number of MDs in Patient Care 20+ hours/wk	Active Licensee, No Restrictions
Data Source:	ASMA (2005)	AMA (2004)	Occ Lic-"AA" with AK address (2005)
MD	1,221	1,347	1,392
DO	92	N/A	109
TOTAL	1,313	1,347	1,501
"Per 1,000"population for the year	1,000 * 1,313/664,000 =1.98	1,000 * 1,347/658,000 =2.05	1,000 * 1501/664,000 =2.26

The Occupational Licensing and ASMA data indicate that 59 percent of Alaska's resident active physicians are based in Anchorage Municipality (including Elmendorf), which accounts for about 42 percent of the State's population. Fifty-one percent of the State's primary care physicians are located in Anchorage. Sixty-eight percent of the State's specialists are in Anchorage.

Physician assistants and advanced nurse practitioners are critical providers of care in Alaska, complementing and extending physician coverage for primary care, for supervision and training of community health aides and practitioners, and in some settings for serving as specialists in surgery, emergency medicine, and other areas. As of the end of 2005, there were 284 active physician assistants with Alaska addresses and "AA" status; 29 percent were in Anchorage. Of 486 advanced nurse practitioners with active licenses and Alaska addresses, 51 percent were in Municipality of Anchorage.

The Task Force used the AMA listing for "physicians in practice" (excluding academics, retirees and others) by specialty, although this is for MDs only. One can be reasonably sure of the validity of comparing Alaska to the U.S. physician to population ratio using this standardized approach. This is the most reliable basis for selecting an "Alaska Standard" for target ratio of physicians (MDs) to population.[10] The physician to population ratio using the AMA count of MDs in patient care 20 hours or more per week is 2.05 physicians per 1,000 population for Alaska for 2004, compared with 2.38 for the United States as a whole. If Alaska had the same number per 1,000 as the United States, there would be 1,569, or 16 percent (218) more physicians in Alaska providing patient care 20 hours per week or more. The current level of 2.05 physicians per 1,000 population puts Alaska 17th lowest among the States.

Keeping in mind the differences among the data sets, and the strengths and limitations of each, summary information is presented from each of the data set as appropriate, to show relevant information about Alaska's physician and mid-level providers. Each data set is useful for specific analyses and comparisons. The data permit examination and consideration of the factors that are likely to influence future demand and supply to 2025.

---

[10] UW Center for Health Workforce Studies Working Paper #98 used the Master File of the AMA to examine age and county distribution of physicians so purchase of the Master File or request to the CHWS could provide for another analysis but this will still be limited to MD degree holders. The licensure and ASMA data sets provide a more complete accounting of Alaska based physicians including Doctors of Osteopathy and physicians not licensed in Alaska but serving in the Public Health Service Commissioned Corps or the Military.

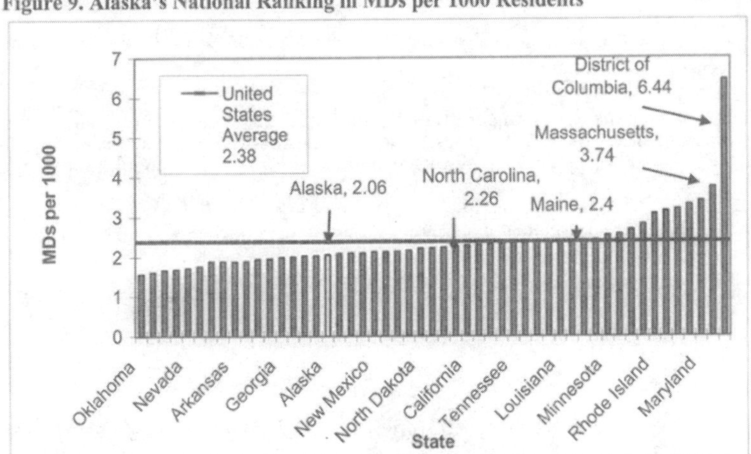

Figure 9. Alaska's National Ranking in MDs per 1000 Residents

Source: AMA 2006

In State rankings of physicians per 1000 population, Alaska's ranking in recent years has varied from sixth lowest to thirty second lowest, depending on whether or not the count includes only non-federal physicians, or whether the ranking focuses on physicians in patient care at least 20 hours per week. Figure 9 shows one method of "ranking" States based on ratios for 2004 counting physicians in patient care.

Alaska has proportionally more "Federal" physicians than most States because of the presence of military physicians, IHS physicians, and Public Health Service Commissioned Corps who serve in several agencies in Alaska. Methods that exclude "Federal" physicians rank Alaska lower in comparisons of "physician to population ratios" because they exclude Federal providers from the numerator, but retain the populations served (military and Alaska Native) in the denominator. (For example, the Kaiser Family Foundation "State health fact" Web site uses the non-federal physician count only.)

Figure 10 shows the numbers of physicians, physician assistants, podiatrists and paramedics licensed by the Alaska State Medical Board. Other data provided below allow for analysis of physicians and mid-level provider counts (including advanced nurse practitioners) in more detail.

Figure 10. Physicians, Podiatrists, Physician Assistants, and Paramedics by Fiscal Year
(licensed regardless of State of residence or practice)

	FY 95	FY 96	FY 97	FY 98	FY 99	FY 00	FY 01	FY 02	FY 03	FY 04	FY 05
MD/DO Active	1,419	1,593	1,603	1,826	1,810	2,034	1,850	2,080	2,099	2,321	2,309
MD/DO Inactive	262	262	277	266	300	289	285	268	249	242	240
Podiatrists Active & Inactive	13	14	14	15	15	16	16	17	18	17	20
Physician Assistants Active & Inactive	200	231	221	255	244	266	245	284	266	297	307
Paramedics-Active	134	158	151	191	195	230	233	255	245	283	280
TOTAL	2,028	2,258	2,266	2,553	2,564	2,835	2,629	2,904	2,877	3,160	3,156

Source: Alaska State Medical Board.

Characteristics of the physician workforce in Alaska. The annual directories from the Alaska State Medical Association and the biennial versions of the Occupational

Licensing database both provide trend information on the following characteristics of physicians [11]:

- demographic characteristics;
- practice characteristics;
- specialty distribution; and
- geographic distribution.

Alaska physicians are younger than the national physician supply, and younger than those in other WWAMI States (average age 48.4 vs. 49.2) according to Chen et al., (Chen, 2005); however as in other States, the physician population is aging.

Figure 11. Alaska Physicians' Age Distribution (MDs)
(N=1580, includes physicians not in practice)

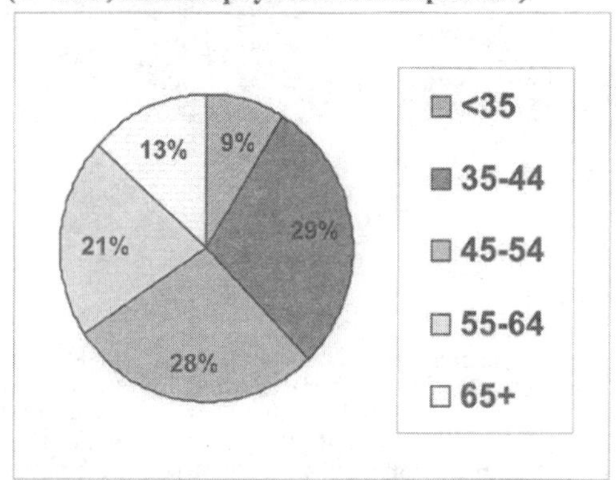

Source: AMA 2006 (from Master File Report for 2004)

Figure 12. US Physicians' Age Distribution (MDs)
(N=884,974, includes physicians not in practice)

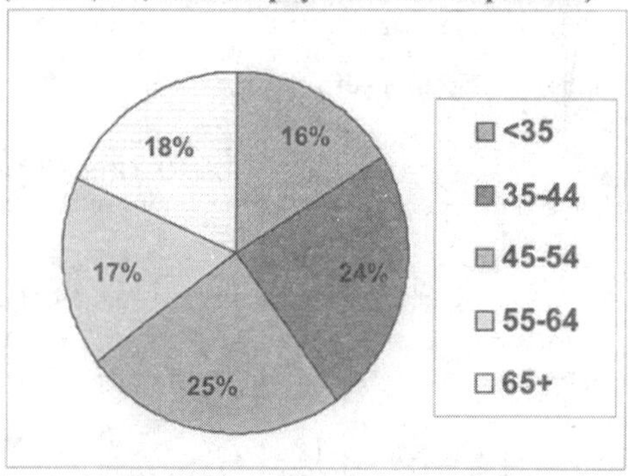

Source: AMA 2006 (from Master File Report for 2004)

Since 1998, the percentages of all physicians who were under age 35, and between 35 and 44 have decreased while the percentages 55 to 64 and 65 and over have increased. However by comparing the ages of those who left Alaska during the 1998–2006 period with those who stayed, one can see that departure rates are similar across age rather than being higher for older physicians.

---

[11] State files: are more current (by a year) than the AMA report (especially useful for military); contain geographic location listed in license application and ASMA membership application; include DOs as well as MDs; provide specialty (ASMA) linked to other characteristics (licensing); allow examination of length of licensure, timing of license applications and license lapses; and allow comparison of licensed providers at different points in time (about every 2 years) to determine approximate age at time of move from Alaska, by specialty; likewise changes in status (locums to regular license, for instance).

Age distribution of physicians (MD and DO), physician assistants and advanced nurse practitioners. As shown in Figures 13 to 15, very few (2 or 3 percent) of advanced nurse practitioners and physician assistants (mid-level providers) are in the age group 65 and older. This compares with 11 percent of physicians being 65 years or older. A proportionally larger number of mid-level practitioners are aged 45–54—about 42 percent compared with 32 percent of physicians.

Figure 13. Age Distribution of Physicians (MDs and DOs) in Alaska N=1501

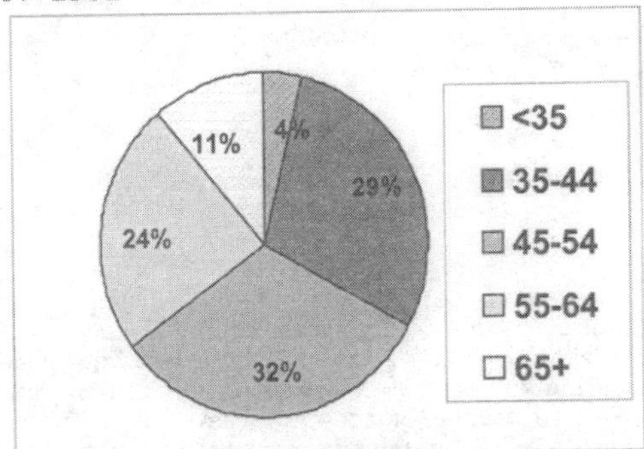

Source: 2006 Alaska Occupational Licensing Database

Figure 14. Age Distribution of Physician's Assistants in Alaska N=294

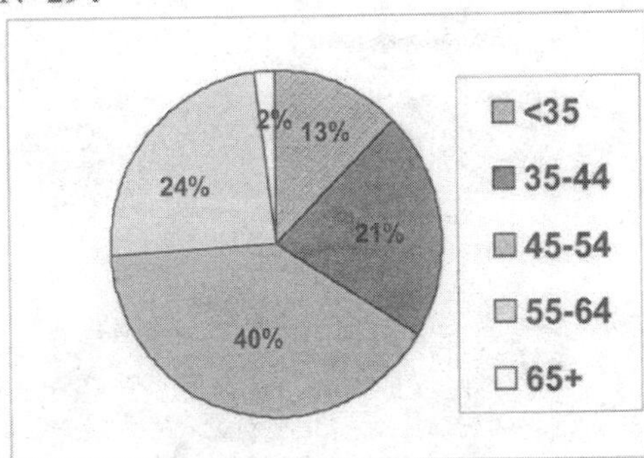

Source 2006 Alaska Occupational Licensing Database

Figure 15. Age Distribution of Advanced Nurse Practitioners in Alaska N= 424

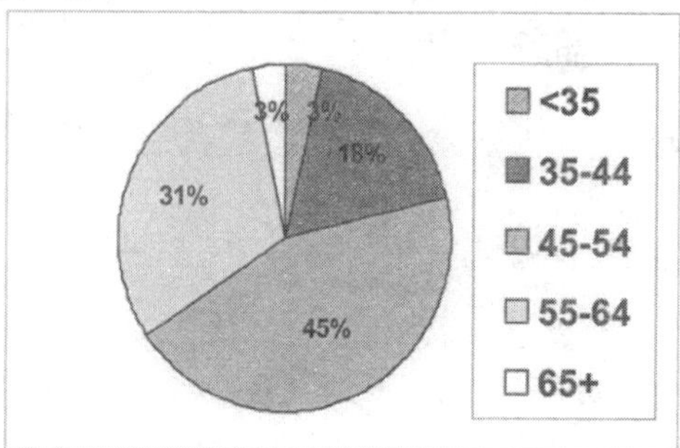

Source: 2006 Alaska Occupational Licensing Database

Figure 16 shows age distribution of both the active physicians in Alaska and the age distribution of those who have let their licenses expire, whose last known address was in Alaska. Some of these individuals may be working in positions that do not require maintenance of an active license, or they may have left the State without informing the State Medical Board. They have 2 years to re-activate their licenses—after that time they need to re-apply for a license.

Figure 16. Age at Expiration of License (Physicians with Most Recent Address in Alaska)

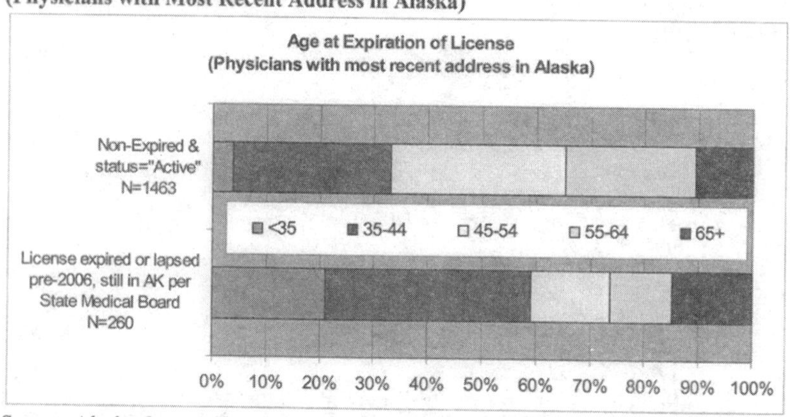

Source: Alaska Occupational Licensing Database analyzed by AKDHSS HPSD

Cohort analysis of the active licensed MDs in 1998 and those who were still active in Alaska as of January 2006 shows a similar age distribution for those who stayed and those who left practice over 8 years (see Figure 17). This suggests that departures from Alaska practice are not predominantly associated with aging and retirement, but occur about equally at any age.

Figure 17. Age of 1998 Cohort "Stayers" and "Leavers"

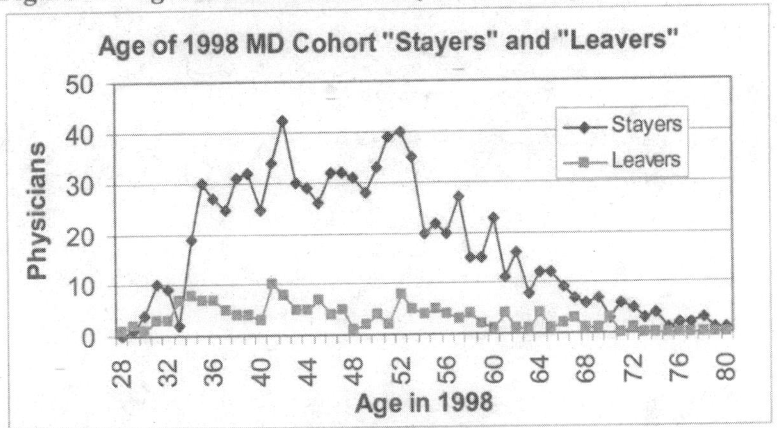

Source: Alaska Occupational Licensing Database analyzed by AKDHSS

Figure 18 compares the age of all physicians who have ever been licensed in Alaska with the number of those who have left the State and no longer hold Alaska licenses. This data again indicates that departures are distributed across all ages, rather than occurring mostly at "retirement" age.

Figure 18. Age at Expiration of License for Non-Current Physicians (Includes out of state and in-state no longer licensed)

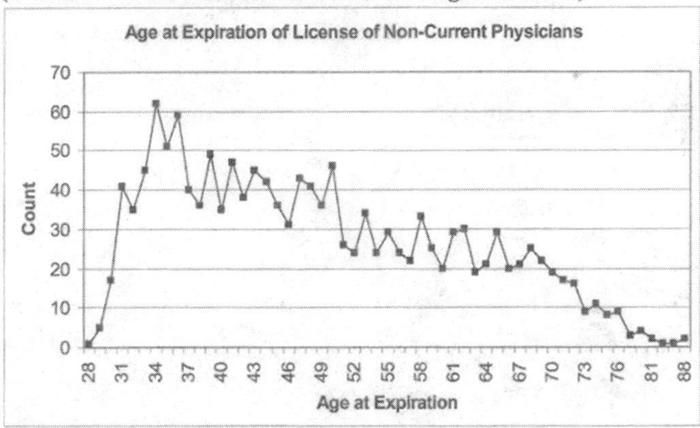

Source: Alaska Occupational Licensing Database analyzed by AKDHSS HPSD

A comparison of active physicians located in Alaska in 2006 and 1998 shows similar age distributions in both groups although the total number of physicians in 2006 is larger (Figure 19, below). It is notable that the number of physicians under age 33 was smaller in 2006 than in 1998, which might suggest failure to recruit recent graduates to the State. With students tending to enter medical school at older ages and taking more years of graduate training, it is likely that this may be true in other States as well, although it appears that only about 9 percent of Alaska's physicians are under age 35, while about 16 percent are under age 35 nationwide. (Figures 11 and 12 above).

Figure 19. Age of Current Active AK Physicians, 2006 & 1998

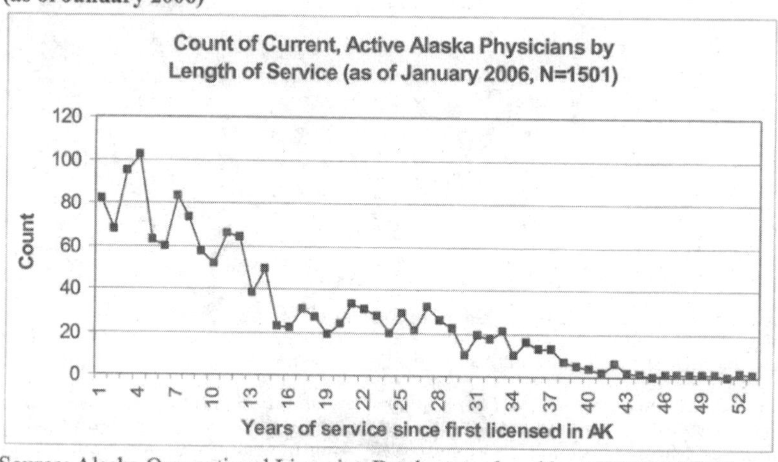

Source: Alaska Occupational Licensing Database analyzed by AKDHSS HPSD

Figure 20 shows length of service for current active physicians living in Alaska, indicating that a very large number and proportion have been in the State for 10 years or less. Retaining current physicians for additional years is a priority for assuring adequate physician supply into the next two decades.

Figure 20. Count of Current, Active AK Physicians by Length of Service (as of January 2006)

Source: Alaska Occupational Licensing Database analyzed by AKDHSS HPSD

New mid-level and physician licensees in Alaska. Graphs of year of entry (year licensed) for current mid-levels and physicians shows that physician assistants are now exceeding advanced nurse practitioners as new licensees, although this is a recent development. Mid-level providers were first licensed in Alaska in 1980. The total of 60 to 70 mid-levels each of the last 2 years approaches the number of new physicians in each of those years (68 and 80), as shown in Figures 21 and 22.

**Figure 21. Alaska Mid-Levels by Type and Year Licensed as of January 1, 2006
(424 NPs & 284 PAs, Total 708, "AA" status, AK residence)**

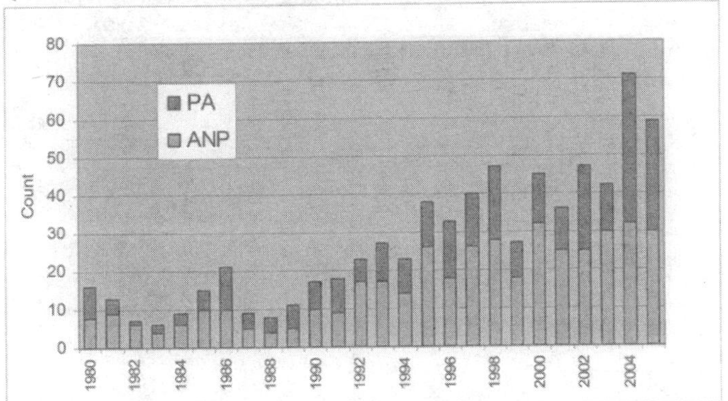

Source: Alaska Occupational Licensing Database analyzed by AKDHSS HPSD

**Figure 22. MDs and DOs by Year Licensed, with License as of January 1, 2006
(1395 MDs, 109 DOs, "AA" status, AK residence)**

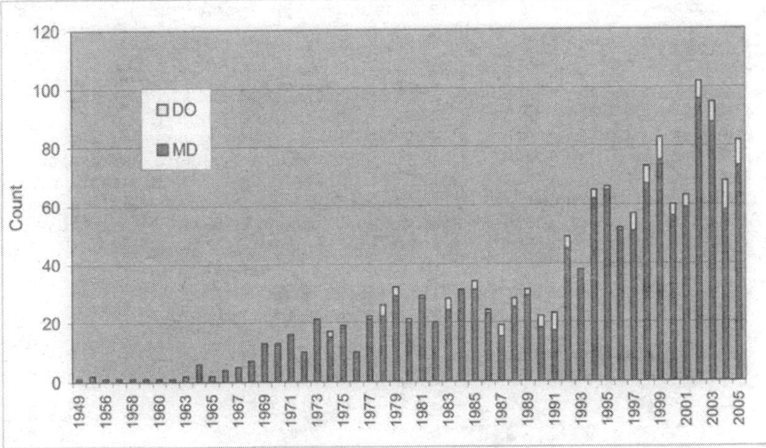

Source: Alaska Occupational Licensing Database analyzed by AKDHSS HPSD

Figure 23 shows the distribution by specialty for allopathic physicians active in patient care (20 hours or more per week), according to the AMA's master file, based on an annual survey. The counts by specialty show that nearly 53 percent of Alaska's allopathic physicians are in primary care, compared with about 50 percent of U.S. physicians being in primary care. Half of Alaska's primary care physicians are family practitioners (366 of 709 primary care physicians), compared with only a third of the Nation's primary care physicians being in family medicine. Nationally, doctors in internal medicine outnumber family practitioners two to one (see Appendix A), while in Alaska the ratio is reversed—there are twice as many family practitioners as internists. For additional data comparing specialty distributions in Alaska and the United States, see Appendix A.

> *"Internal Medicine private practice is part of a dying breed unless something is done. There are many more specialists and sub-specialists than general Internal Medicine physicians in Anchorage now. If our trend continues, there will be few*

or no general Internal Medicine private physicians in Anchorage due to high stu-dent debts and low Medicare payment rates."
—RICHARD NEUBAUER, MD, INTERNAL MEDICINE, ANCHORAGE,
AMERICAN COLLEGE OF PHYSICIANS, BOARD OF REGENTS.

Figure 23. Alaska 2004 Patient Care Physicians (MDs) by Specialty

Specialty	Total Patient Care Physicians 2004 (MDs, per AMA)	Patient Care Physicians per 1000 population	Percent of Total by Specialty or Group (2004)
Total Physicians	1,347	2.05	100
Primary Care	709	1.08	52.6
Family Medicine (& GP)	366	0.56	27.2
Internal Medicine	157	0.24	11.7
Pediatrics	108	0.16	8.0
Ob/Gyn	78	0.12	5.8
Medical Specialties	55	0.08	4.1
Surgical Specialties	237	0.36	17.6
Psychiatry	69	0.10	4.9
Emergency Medicine	72	0.11	5.3
Other Specialties	205	0.31	15.2

Source: AMA Master File

Besides focusing on differing specialties, physicians work in differing practice set-tings, such as private practice, State or municipal or Federal public health activi-ties, and military service. The Alaska State Medical Association surveys its mem-bers regarding their practice settings. Private practice accounts for the vast majority of practice settings (nearly 1,200 physicians). The number of military physicians who have let ASMA know about their presence has shrunk in recent years, account-ing even for a shrinkage in the absolute number of physicians listed in 2004, but the licensing list indicates there was in fact not a decline in active licensed physi-cians. A review of the ASMA listing and occupational licensure found that some physicians working in the Alaska tribal health care systems do not list their names with ASMA. Certain physicians in Federal service may work in the State without an Alaska license. See Figure 24 for the distribution by practice type of physicians in the ASMA databases for 1997 through 2005.

Figure 24. Physicians by Practice Type in Alaska

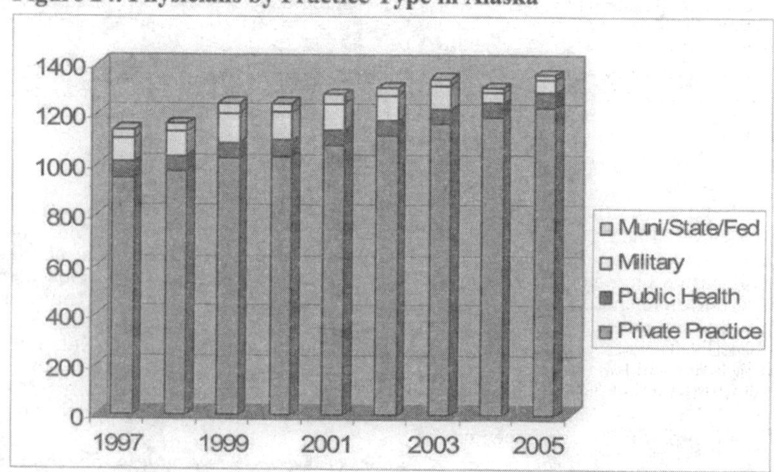

Source: ASMA Directories 1997-2005

Typically some portion of the military physicians have worked part-time in the private sector. Both military and public health service staff detailed to Alaska have served as a rich resource for recruitment into the private and public sector resident physician workforce, according to anecdotal reports.

Forecasting Assumptions. The Physician Supply Task Force agreed on general principles for forecasting need for physicians.

1. Assume that the proportion of physicians whose area of practice is primary care will remain close to the 2004-05 level (53 percent). This proportion is expected to drop up to three points, to 50 percent, as the number of physicians practicing in medical subspecialties such as cardiology and pulmonology, and in psychiatric specialties, which are far below national norms, are brought more into alignment with population needs.

2. Assume that the ratio of DOs to MDs, and the ratios of physician assistants and advanced nurse practitioners licensed to practice in Alaska, will remain the same as the 2004–05 levels. In practice the ratio of DOs to MDs has increased gradually over time to 1:11, while the number of mid-level providers has increased more rapidly than the number of physicians of both types since 1980. The increase may level off unless training programs for mid-levels expand faster than expected.

3. The rationale for estimating "need" for physicians at 110 percent of the national norm is based on several considerations.

a. Rural Alaska communities require a regionalized system. This is operationalized by the Alaska tribal health corporations, which generally staff the smallest village clinics with community health aides and practitioners who will continue to be the primary day-to-day health workforce in those clinics. In the tribal health care system, mid-levels provide care and train and supervise community health aides and practitioners, but physician back up is required for complex and severe cases and for oversight of other providers' services and training. The system requires physician travel and office time for handling phone and telehealth consults, supervision, training, and direct patient care.

b. To attain Continuing Education Units (CEUs) and continuing education for professional development and maintaining licensure, physicians in Alaska require more time for the travel involved than physicians in the "Lower 48." Even if additional full time equivalents (FTE) in patient care are not needed, more individuals may be needed to provide the FTE equivalents.

c. In rural and frontier areas, part-time staff cannot be available on short notice as easily as in urban areas. There is thus a structural "inefficiency" in that a community that may need 1.2 physicians according to national norms will require two physicians, and communities that would be expected to need a fraction of a physician FTE will need to be served either by a mid-level provider, a community health aide or practitioner, or by transporting patients or providers.

d. Although Alaskans are younger than the population of the United States as a whole, Alaskans engage in more high-risk occupational and subsistence activities. Thus Alaska's typical case mix results in higher than average needs of the population.

e. High poverty segments of the population tend to have additional risks associated with both environmental hazards and lifestyle behaviors. Since much of the low-income population is in the most remote parts of the State, this adds to the burden of illness and injury to be addressed in the areas hardest to reach with physician services.

Figure 25. Physician Need Forecasts for 2025

Physicians (MDs) in patient care, 2004:	1,347	2.05 per 1,000 population
2004 MD count if at U.S. norm (2.38)	1,565	2.38 per 1,000 population
Current shortage using U.S. Norm:	(218)	
Current shortage using 110 percent U.S. Norm:	(375)	
2025 MD Need Forecasts:		
U.S. Forecast need for 2025 2.82/1,000 * 1.1 = 3.1 per 1,000.	2,444	3.1 per 1,000 population
Additional Physicains Needed:	1,097	
Average Annual "gain" needed, 21 years:	52	

Figure 26 compares several possible patterns of increase in physician (MD) supply and the "desired gain" linear increase that is based on Alaska reaching the target of 110 percent of the U.S. norm of physicians per 1,000 people by 2025. The "potential access gap" suggests the widening gap between the anticipated need forecast by the Task Force and supply if supply fails to increase. Strategies recommended below aim to ensure that the gap does not widen, and the need for adequate physician supply is met over the next two decades.

Figure 26. Gain in Alaskan Physicians (MDs): Static Doctor to Population Ratio vs. Desired Growth

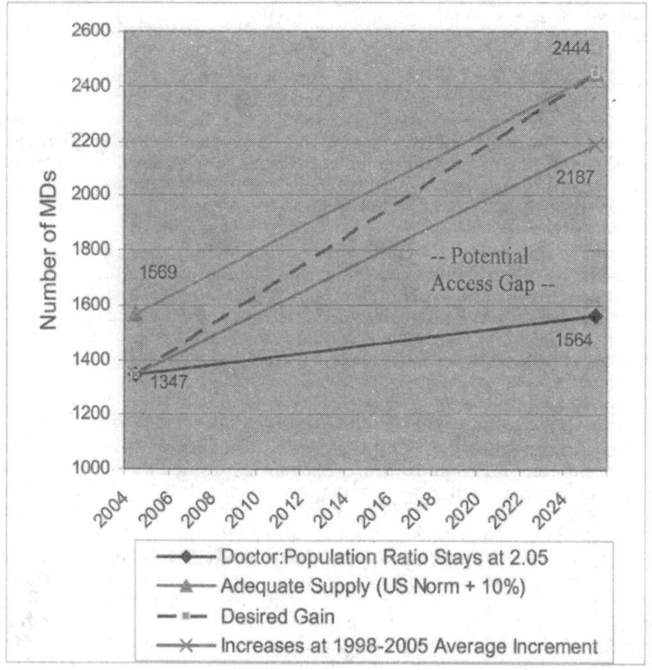

SECTION V. OVERVIEW OF ALASKA'S CURRENT HEALTH CARE WORKFORCE DEVELOPMENT AND TRAINING ACTIVITIES

A. MEDICAL SCHOOL OPPORTUNITIES FOR ALASKANS

"I was first on the waiting list for University of Washington. They only had space for 10 Alaskans and I was 11th, so I went to OHSU in Portland, Oregon. OHSU is not part of the WWAMI program. I paid out-of-state tuition, roughly four times more expensive than the WWAMI program. My intention from the time of my medical school application was to become a family practice physician in Alaska. OHSU was an excellent school, but I had to arrange my own training experiences in Alaska with my elective rotations, one of which was in Dillingham where I now work."
—LEIF THOMPSON, MD. BRISTOL BAY AREA HEALTH CORPORATION.

Wyoming, Washington, Alaska, Montana and Idaho (WWAMI). For the past 35 years Alaska has participated in a unique collaborative medical education program known as the WWAMI Program. In 1971 Alaska was the first State to join with the University of Washington School of Medicine in an initiative designed to provide medical school opportunities in northwest rural States that did not have their own 4-year medical schools. WWAMI decentralizes medical education, allowing medical students to receive training in their home States and in rural settings. This approach encourages students to return to their home States or WWAMI States to practice medicine. WWAMI remains the only in-state medical education opportunity available to Alaskans.

Each year since 1971 there have been 10 medical student slots available for Alaskans in WWAMI. Admission to Alaska WWAMI has become extremely competitive. In 2005–06 there were about eight Alaskan applicants for each slot.

The applicants selected for admission to WWAMI pay in-state tuition rates, about $20,000 less than out-of-state tuition. This $20,000 difference is subject to a payback provision, but is forgiven if the recipient practices in Alaska after medical school. Twenty percent of the total amount is forgiven for each year of practice. The payback provision was enacted in 1999. Its impact cannot yet be assessed, but it is likely to increase the rate of return.

Alaskans who are admitted to WWAMI now complete their first year of medical school at the University of Alaska Anchorage, their second year at the University of Washington, and their third and fourth years in clerkships and rotations in Alaska or other WWAMI locations. Signing up for clerkships and rotations in Alaska is the mechanism that allows for completion of nearly 3 years of the 4-year curriculum in Alaska.

Such clerkships and rotations are partially supported by the Alaska Department of Health and Social Services, the University of Alaska Anchorage, and the University of Washington, most often using federally funded grant programs, so that the students' costs are minimized.

An average of seven to eight WWAMI medical students begins practice in Alaska each year. Five of those students are from the cadre of 10 per year in Alaska WWAMI. The other two or three come from one of the other WWAMI States and are students who usually completed a 3rd or 4th year medical school clerkship experience in Alaska as part of their WWAMI medical education. Figure 27 depicts the effectiveness of the WWAMI affiliations in producing doctors for Alaska. The 50 percent rate of return on Alaska's investments in 10 Alaska medical students ranks it as #5 among all U.S. States (AAMC, 2006).

The WWAMI program as part of the University of Washington School of Medicine is consistently ranked among the very best medical school programs in the United States. The University of Washington is ranked as the #1 primary care medical school in the Nation, for the 14th consecutive year (*The U.S. News and World Report*, 2006). It was also ranked first in family medicine and rural medicine, and in the top 10 in every category that was ranked. Thus, WWAMI offers a superior medical education to Alaskans while providing that education largely in-state, encouraging students to return to practice and helping to build in-state capacity.

Figure 27. WWAMI Outcomes Flow Chart

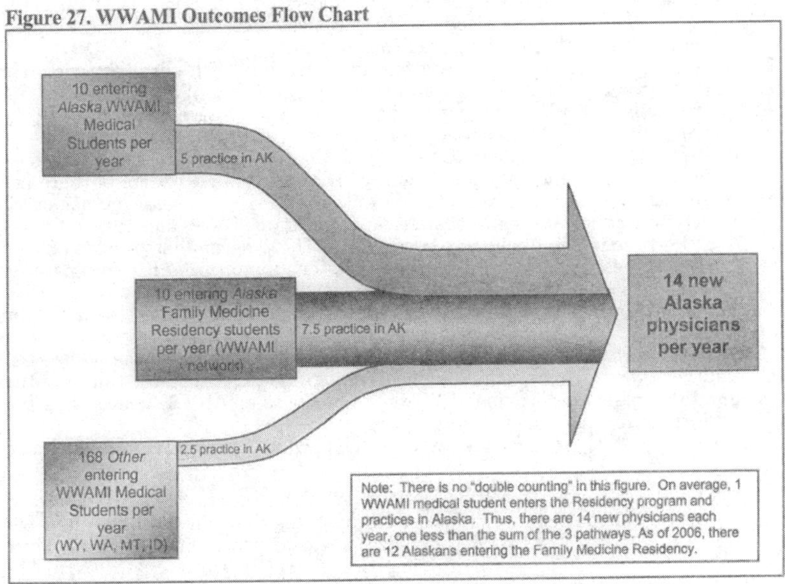

Source: D. Valenzeno, personal communication

"We have such an exceptional applicant pool for our 10 Alaska WWAMI slots. Last year, all applicants had very strong grade point averages and MCAT scores. The number of slots that we have in WWAMI has not increased to reflect the needs of our growing and aging population."
—PETER MARSHALL, MD. PRIVATE PRACTICE, NORTH POLE.

Western Interstate Commission on Higher Education (WICHE). In the past, the WICHE program has provided access to medical education (including osteopathy) and other fields of graduate or professional study for the residents of member states. The WICHE PSEP provided preferential admissions consideration (above other non-resident applicants) in participating institutions in the participating States, and in doing so agreed to charge admitted PSEP students either the resident tuition rate, or, for those private institutions participating, a reduced rate of tuition. In return, the State "sending" the participant agreed to pay a support fee associated with each of its residents in the program. However, the program for students of medicine and osteopathy ended in 1997, after supporting 528 student years of study for medical students, 82 of whom were in osteopathic medicine between 1982 and 1997, at a cost of $5,700,000. The unduplicated student count was 176 (Barrans Memo, 2006). The "return rate" for WICHE-supported students is reported to be 18 percent, which means the program supported about 35 physicians who have served in Alaska.

B. Graduate Medical Education in Alaska—the Alaska Family Medicine Residency

Alaska's only in-state GME program is the AFMR. Alaska was the last State in the United States to have a residency program. The AFMR was developed in the 1990s by a consortium of State health leaders with the intent to train family physicians for the unique aspects of practice in the most remote parts of the State. AFMR residents receive extra training in emergency medicine, orthopedics, obstetrics, pediatrics, neonatal intensive care, and trans-cultural medicine to prepare them for the exigencies of bush practice.

The AFMR program started in 1997 with eight residents per class, and expanded to ten residents per year in 2004 and twelve in 2006. Since AFMR's first graduating class in 2000, the program has graduated a total of 55 physicians. Of these graduates 70 percent remain in Alaska to practice after graduation. This gives Alaska the highest rate of return for GME in the United States (AAMC, 2006). Fifty-five percent of them practice in rural communities and one-third practice in tribal health corporation facilities.[12]

The AFMR residents are drawn from the Alaska WWAMI program and other medical schools throughout the United States and other countries. They all arrive with the expressed interest in practicing in rural settings and most of them have a commitment to Alaska from the start of their training.

AFMR program faculty members are family physicians with rural experience in Alaska and other parts of the United States. The program's affiliation with the University of Washington WWAMI program provides for faculty development and access to academic resources which otherwise would not be available in Alaska.

The Providence Family Medicine Center is the outpatient clinic where residents in the program receive much of their training. The faculty and residents there provide comprehensive primary care including outpatient visits, disease management, health maintenance, hospital care, obstetrical care and delivery, and surgical procedures for all corners in the Anchorage community. The program has provided 30,000 patient visits per year with over 15 percent of its population from low-income uninsured.

The AFMR has operated at a deficit since its inception because of several factors unique to Alaska.

1. Most funding for resident training is provided by Medicare through the GME funding authority, and this revenue is 25 percent to 50 percent lower than in other States due to a smaller proportion of Medicare business at AFMR's sponsoring hospital, Providence Alaska Medical Center.

2. The average reimbursement per visit is below what many other residencies experience.

3. Unlike most States, the State of Alaska does not appropriate State general funds for direct support of the residency program. The State of Alaska does support the Residency through Medicaid, as do most States, by reimbursing the hospital for Medicaid's share of the costs of the program, (about $875,000 per year) and by paying full-Medicaid-rate professional fees for the medical care rendered by the program to Medicaid patients in the Providence Family Medicine Center and the hospital (about $668,000 per year).

---

[12]This is an exceptional result compared to residencies in other States. Even the best rural training programs consider themselves very successful if they can place 40 percent of their graduates in rural communities.

C. State, Federal and Tribal Efforts to Support Health Care Workforce Development

State, Federal and tribal funds support an array of health care workforce development and training activities that are critical to improved access and quality of care in Alaska. There are programs for health career development, pre-med programs, loan repayment programs, placement programs for medical student rotations, and recruitment and retention programs that encourage health workforce growth. Alaska placements and sites are not, however, always available to interested applicants.

Health career development. Although not focused strictly on preparing and guiding qualified students into the practice of medicine, new curriculum offerings not available a decade ago provide more educational choices to Alaskan students, and these can lead to heightened interest in medical careers. The University of Alaska has expanded its nursing program and added courses in basic sciences, nutrition, public health, behavioral health, biology, and other health-related subjects, as well as a health sciences major for undergraduates and Masters in Public Health program for graduate students, all of which provide opportunities for preparation for health careers.

In 2005, the University of Alaska Anchorage's School of Nursing received funds from HRSA to establish a basic AHEC program. Nationwide, the AHEC program creates formal relationships between universities and community partners to strengthen the health workforce in underserved communities. For Alaska, community partners developed in the first 3 years of funding are the Yukon Kuskokwim Health Corporation AHEC Center (serving YK Delta region) and Fairbanks Memorial Hospital AHEC Center (serving Fairbanks and the Interior) and the Alaska Family Practice Residency AHEC Center (serving the Anchorage and the Mat-Su Borough). The Alaska AHEC network achieves its collective purpose by encouraging Alaska's youth to pursue careers in health care, facilitating clinical rotation opportunities in underserved sites, and improving access to continuing education for health professionals in underserved areas.

The University of Alaska WWAMI Program offers a high school summer enrichment program called the Della Keats/U-DOC Summer Enrichment Program. The goal of this program is to foster, affirm, and encourage high school students' interest in the medical professions by allowing them to explore health careers and to obtain a valuable introduction to college life. Applicants must be Alaska residents with a strong interest in the health professions. Underrepresented minority, rural-area, first-generation, and/or economically disadvantaged students are encouraged to apply. Stipends may be available to help with the costs of participating in this program.

As well as the University of Alaska, the ANTHC administers several programs that focus on health career development. The ANTHC Education and Development Department awards five scholarships of $5,000 per academic year in health care-related fields to full-time undergraduate students and five scholarships of $5,000 per academic year in health care-related fields to full-time graduate students who are Alaska Native or American Indian permanent Alaska residents. ANTHC grants these scholarships as an integral part of its long-term strategy of providing the highest quality health care services to all Alaska Natives and American Indians. ANTHC graduate scholarships provide supplemental funds for graduate education for students with the greatest demonstrated need.

ANTHC works with the IHS to administer a scholarship program. The IHS Scholarship provides selected scholarship recipients who are Alaska Native or American Indian permanent Alaska residents with paid tuition, related fees, a small amount for travel and books, and a monthly stipend for living expenses. IHS currently funds several health career and allied health career scholarship programs.

The ANTHC runs a summer internship program that awards 9-week paid internships to approximately 25 high school and undergraduate students and five graduate students who are Alaska Native or American Indian permanent Alaska residents. ANTHC grants these internships as part of its long-term strategy of providing the highest quality health services to all Alaska Natives and American Indians and providing work experience in a range of medical professions and support services.

> *"I completed my undergraduate studies at Cornell and came out of college with no debt. I went to medical school at Yale and fell in love with Internal Medicine. I took an IHS scholarship for medical school, which led to my 2-year position in Wyoming. I completed my residency in Michigan. I worked in Juneau for 6 months and am now in private practice in Anchorage. The amount of debt that medical students now accrue is problematic. Since I had not incurred significant*

student debts, it never occurred to me to consider going into a high pay specialty."
—RICHARD NEUBAUER, MD. INTERNAL MEDICINE, ANCHORAGE,
AMERICAN COLLEGE OF PHYSICIANS, BOARD OF REGENTS.

Medical student clinical experiences. Medical students have the opportunity to have clinical experience in Alaska's clinical sites at the end of the first year of medical school. Most of the programs discussed here focus on rural sites. All of these programs give priority to students that are either residents of Alaska or have some ties to the State. This approach is based on evidence that students who are trained in rural areas tend to work in rural areas and that that they tend to work near their training sites. Thus, it is anticipated that they are more likely to return to the State to attend the AFMR or to serve as physicians after graduation.

Alaska has at least three programs that provide clinical experiences or medical student clinical rotations in the State. The Department of Health and Social Services (Alaska Primary Care Office) administers the NHSC Student/Resident Experiences and Rotations in Community Health (NHSC SEARCH) program, also called the Alaskan Exposure program. The ANTHC places students and residents in rotations in tribal sites. The Alaska Center for Rural Health (ACRH) manages the Rural/Underserved Opportunities Program (R/UOP) summer clinical experience for WWAMI students in Alaska.

The NHSC SEARCH: Alaskan Exposure program supports rotations for an average of 40 health professions students each year in underserved sites. Of these 40 health professions students, about 20 per year are medical students and residents. This program gives priority to Alaska residents and NHSC scholarship recipients, and also places interested medical students and residents from throughout the United States. It also partners with the AFMR, the R/UOP program, and the ANTHC to support rotations for medical students and residents.

The ANTHC supports several rotations in IHS sites each year for fourth-year medical students and medical residents who apply and are accepted from schools throughout the United States. The Rural/Underserved Opportunities Program, administered by the ACRH, supports rotations each year for students who have just completed their first year at the University of Washington School of Medicine (WWAMI program).

Scholarship and loan repayment programs. Some physicians take positions in Alaska through a Federal scholarship or loan repayment program with a service obligation. Such programs in Alaska include the NHSC and the IHS. NHSC scholars can meet their scholarship obligation by working at underserved sites with high federally designated Health Professional Shortage Area (HPSA) scores. Since most Alaskan sites with high enough HPSA scores are too small to support physicians, the placement opportunities are very limited, resulting in only a few physician recruits for Alaska through this program.

The Alaska Primary Care Office (APCO) works with Alaska sites and the Federal Government to conduct research for federally designated HPSAs and, with other State PCOs, seeks to make the HPSA process more effective in identifying areas experiencing difficulty in filling positions, where the need for additional health professionals may be acute but not reflected in physician to population ratios. The APCO also serves as HRSA's designated lead contact to link interested NHSC physicians with Alaska sites, thereby supporting the recruitment of these physicians.

Placement at Alaska sites through the NHSC loan repayment program is more extensive than through NHSC scholarship obligations because NHSC has not required such high HPSA scores for loan repayment. Under the loan repayment program a physician works for 2 years at a qualified HPSA site in exchange for up to $25,000 of loan repayment, tax-free, with the option to renew year by year for up to $35,000 per year. Currently there are eight NHSC physician loan repayers working in Alaska. Physician specialties eligible for NHSC support are family medicine, general pediatrics, general internal medicine, general psychiatry, and obstetrics/gynecology.

Alaska is one of 13 States that does not participate in the HRSA Bureau of Health Professions State Loan Repayment Program. Funding for this program is matched 50/50 by NHSC. The APCO and others have researched and coordinated efforts to organize one of these programs for Alaska and gain the required 50 percent State match, but funds have not been identified. In this program NHSC grants matching funds directly to States to operate their own loan repayment programs. Primary care health professionals who are providing full-time clinical services in a public or non-profit facility located in a federally designated Health Professional Shortage Area are eligible for this program. Eligibility requirements and benefits vary from State to State.

The IHS has several scholarship programs to support health education. Some require a service obligation at a qualified IHS site. Under the IHS loan repayment program, applicants sign contractual agreements for 2 years and fulfill their agreements through full-time clinical practice at an IHS facility or approved Alaska Native tribal health program. In return, the loan repayment program will repay all or a portion of the applicant's eligible health professionals educational loans (undergraduate and graduate) for tuition expenses. Applicants are eligible to have their educational loans repaid in amounts up to $20,000 per year for each year of service, tax-free. Eligible specialties are family medicine, internal medicine, pediatrics, geriatric medicine, obstetrics and primarily gynecology, and podiatric medicine. Currently there are 18 IHS physician loan repayers working in Alaska.

"As far as scholarships, there is very little available. I couldn't find any scholarships while in medical school. I was able to find enough funding in loans to cover my tuition and living expenses, roughly $50,000/year, but most of these were unsubsidized loans. In general the more you have to borrow, the less attractive the loans, and the greater the loan fees. I considered National Health Service Corps, however there were very few sites for service in Alaska. I didn't want to risk having to work outside of Alaska to fulfill a commitment."
—LEIF THOMPSON, MD. BRISTOL BAY AREA HEALTH CORPORATION.

Recruitment and retention. Several organizations provide some support for the recruitment of physicians in Alaska. These organizations focus primarily on their own mandates and specific grant requirements. The ANTHC provides recruitment and referral service and support to tribally managed hospitals and clinics throughout Alaska. The Alaska Primary Care Association (APCA) maintains an updated list of *locum tenens* providers and a clearinghouse of candidates looking for permanent opportunities in Alaska's Community Health Centers. The Northwest Regional Primary Care Association has instituted a fee-for-service recruitment service to Alaska sites. The Alaska Department of Labor has a job bank for vacancies in health care settings.

The APCO coordinates some placement efforts, provides recruitment and retention training, researches Health Professional Shortage Areas, and analyzes workforce need. The APCO also serves as a focal point for NHSC activities, providing technical assistance to monitor and increase the number of sites and individuals qualified for NHSC.

The Alaska Office of Rural Health in DHSS supports recruitment and retention by strengthening Alaska's rural health system, facilitating network development and administering Alaska's State Web page on the Rural Recruitment and Retention Network (3RNET) Web site, where clinical sites can advertise positions and health care workers can seek jobs. There is no charge to sites or job seekers for this service. The posting of positions on 3RNet does not include in-depth candidate screening, this function is the responsibility of the site recruiting the provider.

Many of Alaska's medicine-related professional associations and membership organizations provide workforce and/or recruitment assistance to their members. As examples, the Alaska State Medical Association, the ASHNA, and the APCA provide guidance and recruitment assistance to their members.

The APCA is a non-profit membership organization founded in 1995 to promote, expand, and optimize access to primary care in Alaska, particularly for the underserved. The APCA works with the private and public sectors to support and connect the organizations and people who provide that care. The APCA promotes workforce development by enhancing internship and rotation opportunities in Alaskan health centers; marketing health center opportunities to students, faculty and alumni; and focusing on retention efforts. With State and Federal partners, the APCA maintains an updated list of *locum tenens* providers and a clearinghouse of candidates looking for permanent opportunities in Alaska.

Alaska recruits some international medical graduates through the J-1 Visa program, which provides incentives to those from other countries to receive their medical education and work as physicians with underserved populations in the United States. The Alaska Primary Care Office coordinates communication for those seeking J-1 visa placements through the United States. Department of State Conrad 30 program. Currently five J-1 physicians serve in Alaska under this program; all are specialists. There were concerns among Task Force members that the J-1 program disadvantages health care delivery in developing countries. More stringent J-1 Visa policies are likely to be enacted which will decrease the physician supply from this source.

According to Task Force members' observations, many physicians have been recruited through the Public Health Service Commissioned Corps and the military. Both entities have undergone system-wide reorganizations and enacted changes to their physician placement policies resulting in reductions to the number of doctors now available to practice medicine in Alaska, and smaller cohorts from which to recruit former military physicians.

The Alaska Department of Health and Social Services contracted with the University of Alaska, ACRH, for a report called the *Status of Recruitment Resources and Strategies*. This report documents that Alaska relies heavily on recruitment to meet its physician workforce needs. Competition for the supply of physicians is dramatically increasing recruitment costs and decreasing return on investment. Between 2004 and 2006, physician recruitment costs in rural Alaska increased nearly 30 percent, from $2,400,000 to $3,400,000. In spite of the scope and cost of these efforts, positions are difficult to fill and physician turnover is high. Physician locum spending nearly tripled between 2004 ($871,000) and 2006 (over $2,300,000) (DHSS/ACRH, 2006).

Workforce development research and infrastructure. The Alaska Primary Care Office (APCO) in the Department of Health and Social Services (DHSS) addresses health care access and workforce disparities that exist in Alaska through the expansion of new access points and the support of existing health centers. The APCO's goals include: assessment of needs; sharing data; workforce development; safety net/ health center growth initiative; designation applications for HPSA and Medically Underserved Areas (MUA); and community development. The APCO is the major point of contact in Alaska for the NHSC, HPSA designations, site development, and students' community-based rotations through the NHSC SEARCH: Alaskan Exposure program.

Between 2000 and 2005, $148,000,000 in Federal funding has been made available through the Denali Commission to support rural health care infrastructure development. As a result, a combined total of 55 clinics have been either built or remodeled and outfitted with quality medical equipment to date. These efforts have improved the physician practice environment, which has aided recruitment efforts. Federal Section 330 funds for community health centers' operations have also supported the rural health care delivery system, resulting in opportunities to staff the clinics. Thus more health centers now offer physician-level staffing to complement mid-levels and community health aides and practitioners.

Alaska has a history that demonstrates its commitment to reducing workforce deficits by establishing innovative programs and leveraging resources. For over 35 years, community health aides and community health practitioners have been providing primary health care in rural Alaska Native villages as the first link in the Alaska tribal health care system. In addition, Alaska has a well-established effective patient care model using mid-levels throughout the State. Utilization of advanced nurse practitioners, physician assistants and community health aides has been a critical component of delivering primary care health care service in Alaska, especially in the most rural regions of the State.

D. Lessons From Other States and From National Studies

Information from other States and national studies point to three types of interventions as being effective in improving physician supply: medical education strategies to address the training experiences of physicians; applicant pool strategies to target the types of students who enter medical school; and practice-environment strategies to make practice more attractive (Grumbach, et al., 1999). Examples of each of these three types of intervention are discussed in several State and national reports as described below. These reports mostly focus on shortages in rural areas. It should be noted that physician shortages also adversely affect access to primary care in urban settings.

Medical education strategies. Kentucky's short-term strategies for addressing physician shortages include increasing State support of Kentucky's residency programs, maintaining or increasing Federal support of rural GME through Medicare and Title VII of the Public Health Service Act. Long-term strategies include expanding rural residency programs to graduate more residents, opening new schools, creating a new residency program in a rural area that needs it most, increasing class size in existing medical schools, and taking steps to increase the "rural pipeline" (Casey, et al., 2004).

Policies that alter the composition of the classes entering medical school have the most delayed effects on service in shortage areas, but are critical elements of a comprehensive plan for addressing the physician shortage because they increase the number of physicians who could practice in medically underserved communities. In California it was recommended to increase resources for science enrichment programs targeted toward K–12 student and college-level educational enrichment programs that focus on promoting interest in the health professions among disadvantaged students. Characteristics that students bring to medical school, such as rural upbringing, racial and ethnic identity, or values of public service, are probably the greatest influences on their decision to practice in an underserved community. Minority physicians are much more likely to practice in underserved communities, and physicians who grew up in rural areas are much more likely to practice in rural communities (Grumbach, et al., 1999).

A Utah study discussed the steps to alleviate physician shortage that included continuing to expand residency training programs as the population grows, to increase rural training, rotations and tracks during residency training, and to increase GME funding this study recommended targeting students most likely to remain in practice and recruiting to increase retention (Taylor, p. 2).

Utah's GME planning initiative may be a model for other States, especially those with only one or two medical schools and a small number of teaching hospitals. Nevada and Hawaii have begun to emulate the model. The goal of the demonstration is to use a portion of the GME monies to increase the number of physicians who choose to practice in rural areas. This funding arrangement has helped increase the number of generalist physicians, particularly in rural and inner city communities (Taylor, p. 2–3).

Increasing medical school capacity, graduate medical training capacity, and medical education and training in shortage areas are key strategies to address California's projected physician shortage (Center for Health Workforce Studies, December, 2004). The supply of rural physicians is largely dependent on the production of family physicians, both allopathic and osteopathic physicians. Although many factors such as rural upbringing, medical school attended and special educational service experiences are important, the final common pathway for the largest number of rural physicians is a family medicine residency (Council on Graduate Medical Education, 1998. p. 23).

The Physician Shortage Area Program (PSAP) at Jefferson Medical College in Philadelphia selectively admits students from rural areas. According to the Director of the PSAP since 1976, graduates of PSAP were eight times more likely to choose rural practice (Wisconsin Hospital Association and the Wisconsin Medical Society, 2004).

Hands-on experiences in underserved communities stimulate and reinforce interest in caring for underserved populations (Grumbach, et al., 1999). The following are examples of clinical rotation programs at State universities. These programs aim to support recruitment and retention of rural physicians. Eight Michigan State University medical students are selected each year for the Rural Physician Program that provides rich clinical experiences and community service opportunities in small towns in order to boost recruitment of rural physicians. University of Illinois College of Medicine Rural Medical Education Program is designed to prepare students for unique challenges that face rural physicians, with a 30-month ambulatory primary care experience at rural primary care centers. Fourth year students participate in a 16-week rural preceptorship in small, rural communities (Wisconsin Hospital Association and the Wisconsin Medical Society, 2004).

Many other States fund GME in part with Medicaid dollars. Federal law allows Medicaid to fund GME through a number of different models, including paying hospitals for direct and indirect GME costs and by increasing the Medicaid payment rate for patient services rendered by teaching physicians and teaching centers, such as the Family Medicine Center. The amount allowed is limited by the Federal Medicare payment amounts. The advantage of maximizing funding through Medicaid is that State appropriations for GME are matched by Federal funds at the Medicaid match rate of at least 1:1.

In addition to supporting Medicaid GME for residencies, many States also appropriate funds directly for their support. An excellent example is the State of Washington program, which supports each of its family medicine programs with about $250,000 per residency per year.

Recruitment strategies. A national study assessed all State programs that provided financial support to medical students, residents and practicing physicians in exchange for a period of service in underserved areas. Compared to younger nonobligated physicians, physicians serving obligations to State programs were more satisfied and remained in their practices longer, half of them staying over 8 years. Retention rates were highest for loan repayment, direct incentive, and loan programs. An advantage of these programs is that they target physicians at the end of their training, when they know more about their career interests, job options, and family needs (Pathman, et al., 2004).

A report on Kentucky's physician shortage identified a number of barriers to physician recruitment and retention, including medical education costs, workload and demands, and decreased opportunity for professional contacts in medically underserved areas. Economic concerns that affected recruitment and retention included publicly supported insurance programs Medicaid and Medicare that reimburse rural providers at a lower rate than urban providers for the same medical procedures; rise in insurance payments; relief coverage and assurance of a reasonable amount of time off from work is the most important factor in decisions to stay or leave. Other issues include quality of public schools and ability to become a part of the local community, which was scored as more important than income. Having an unhealthy population with high rates of disease including heart disease, hypertension, asthma, diabetes and cancer can adversely affect the ability to recruit and retain physicians. Kentucky's short-term strategies for addressing physician workforce shortages include creating waivers for physician placement in rural areas, allowing alternative loan repayment matching funds, using coal severance tax returns for State match for the SLRP, using physician placement services, and continuing support of J-1 visa waivers (Casey, et al., 2004).

A study about California's physician shortage recommended increasing the diversity of the physician workforce, and providing incentives to encourage physicians to migrate to the State as well as incentives to retain physicians currently practicing in the State (Center for Health Workforce Studies, December, 2004).

Physicians whose spouses are from urban areas stay in practice as long as those whose spouses are from rural areas. Length of stay in rural practice is not associated with attending a public vs. private medical school or with training in a community-based vs. medical school-based residency. Physicians involved in teaching remain in rural practice longer than those who are not involved. For obligated NHSC scholars, students from private schools are more likely to stay in a rural payback site after they have fulfilled their obligation period than are those from public medical schools. Although many urban physicians assume otherwise, rural physicians do not necessarily view professional isolation and an inability to access medical information as drawbacks to rural practice. Lack of quality of rural school systems, perceived or real, is related to length of stay for physicians in a rural practice (American Academy of Family Physicians, 2006.)

The location of a physician's training influences his or her future choices of practice location. Students with rural origins are more likely to train in primary care and return to rural areas; however, they are no more likely to stay in rural practice than are those who were raised in urban areas. Residents who have their training in rural areas are more likely to choose to practice in rural areas. Family medicine is the key discipline of rural health care. Residents practice close to where they train (Council on Graduate Medical Education, 1998).

Community and health care leaders must acknowledge that their communities may not have the economic capacity to support physicians or maintain state-of-the-art equipment and facilities. This situation can be caused by low population of the community, high poverty status of the community, or because the community is too geographically isolated or disadvantaged to financially support physicians. Continuous subsidies would be required to sustain a physician in such areas (Wright, et al., 2001).

Practice environment strategies. Strategies offered to meet California's physician shortage included the following: increase the productivity and capacity of the existing physician workforce through expansion of the supply and use of non-physician clinicians, investment in new technologies, increasing the use of treatment protocols and utilization review. Promoting physician loan repayment and placement programs are key strategies noted in a study addressing California's shortages (Center for Health Workforce Studies, December, 2004).

Regarding practice environment, it was recommended that California: (1) resurrect its Shortage Area Medical Matching Program which matched graduating residents with practice opportunities in underserved areas; (2) match Federal funding for the NHSC SLRP; (3) support pilot programs that encourage innovative public health-oriented prevention activities for physicians participating in the above programs; and (4) support the Rural/Underserved Provider Opportunity Program's *locum tenens* network in rural California (Grumbach, et al., 1999).

In addition to examples from California that address the physician practice environment, a Kentucky study recommended reforming medical liability as a means of improving the practice environment (Casey, et al., 2004).

Workforce planning. A workforce report focused on California recommended promoting a more effective environment for physician workforce planning and policies through increasing data collection and monitoring around physician requirements, developing systems to track physician supply and requirements, comprehensive reassessment of physician supply and requirements every 5 years, and establishing an overall statewide process for physician workforce planning (Center for Health Workforce Studies, December, 2004).

Strategies included in a Utah report were developing a Comprehensive State Health Care Workforce Plan to coordinate the training of various health professions and maximize limited State resources, i.e., funding, faculty and infrastructure, prioritizing statewide needs by specialty, and improving data collection methods for ongoing collection of physician data (Taylor, p. 2–3). A national shortage affects the supply of physicians in Utah; they can no longer rely on the national pool to cover local deficits (Taylor, p. 2–3).

"Steps should be taken to build stronger rural health communities that mobilize all types of human resources (e.g., patients and family care givers) and institutions (e.g., educational, social, and faith-based) to both augment and support the contributions of health professionals." (Committee on the Future of Rural Health Care, 2005, Chapter 4).

Key strategies to address California's projected physician shortages include promoting programs and policies to address physician mal-distribution by region and specialty, offering targeted site development grants, and increasing reimbursement rates in shortage areas (Center for Health Workforce Studies, December, 2004).

The NHSC Site Development Manual includes a chapter on "Involving the Community" (U.S. DHHS, 2006). This manual recommends the formation of Community Primary Health Care Councils that will be involved in making decisions related to the community's health care system, including developing sites that can tap into NHSC resources and providers who are NHSC Scholars or are eligible for NHSC Loan Repayment.

SECTION VI. CLOSING THE GAP: STRATEGIES FOR "GROWING OUR OWN"—TRAINING, RECRUITING, AND RETAINING PHYSICIANS FOR ALASKA

A. CONTEXT AND PROCESS FOR SELECTION OF STRATEGY RECOMMENDATIONS

One of the two primary charges to the Alaska Physician Task Force was to identify strategies that could address the need for physicians in Alaska over the next 25 years. In order to formulate its response to this charge, the Task Force collected its findings regarding the need for physicians and the nature of physician supply, along with previous strategies in both Alaska and other States.

From March 2006 through July 2006, the Task Force and staff undertook a detailed investigation of various strategies that have been in place in Alaska and other States. The Task Force engaged experts in Alaska, the University of Washington, and others outside the State, and reviewed literature from national and professional organizations. Also considered were physician supply data and trends, Alaska population demographic predictions, physician recruitment and retention experience in Alaska and other States, current physician practice environment, and the professional experience of those consulted during the deliberations.

Beginning with about forty potential strategies gleaned from their research, the Task Force reviewed and rated each strategy according to feasibility, cost, desirability, effectiveness, and length of time that the strategy would take to affect Alaska's physician supply, and then concluded with a shorter list of recommended strategies and action steps for this report. The list of the original strategies and their ratings is in Appendix B.

The Task Force's selections of strategies are based on the following findings:

Finding 7. Alaska is one of six States without an independent in-state medical school. Alaska funds 10 state-supported "seats" at the regional WWAMI medical school, administratively centered at the University of Washington School of Medicine. This number (10 seats) represents fewer seats per capita than all but 5 of the 50 States.

Finding 8. Residency programs are one of the most effective ways to produce physicians for a State or community. Alaska has only one in-state residency, the AFMR, which places 70 percent of its graduates in Alaska. Maintaining and expanding residency opportunities will be critical in augmenting Alaska's physician numbers.

Finding 9. Over the last 10 years, an increasing number of Alaskan students have applied to medical schools; the average number of applicants has been 65. In 2005, 29 of 73 applicants were admitted into medical school. Ten per year attend WWAMI and the remainder attends medical schools without State support from Alaska. Since 1996, only WWAMI has had Alaska-supported seats. Prior to 1996, Alaska supported programs for medical and osteopathic students through the WICHE program and student loans.

Finding 10. Recruitment for physicians is facilitated by the availability of loan repayment programs such as the IHS and NHSC loan repayment programs. Service obligations related to student loans have historically accounted for some recruitment and should be explored.

Finding 11. There are several initiatives to increase interest in medical careers among Alaskans, including efforts by the tribal health care system, hospitals, the University of Alaska's newly funded AHEC and the UA Scholars Awards, school system initiatives for improvement of math and science programs, and programs that encourage students to go into health careers. Collectively, these initiatives generate qualified applicants to medical schools, but too few applicants matriculate to replenish Alaska's shortage, and there is inadequate diversity.

Finding 12. Medical practice environments in Alaska have positive and negative aspects that affect the recruitment and retention of physicians.

Finding 13. Surveys of providers (physicians and mid-levels) by the AMA and many States have provided data on practice characteristics, preferences, and retirement plans.

Finding 14. Workforce development activities exist in multiple locations including the tribally managed system, private sector, and various State and Federal agencies. However existing programs are not monitoring or analyzing specialty distribution or needs, changing roles of mid-level providers, or potential impact of electronic health records on all providers. Coordination of the efforts, and research and analysis of relevant trends, should inform policy.

The Task Force recognized that forecasting physician supply and need is a daunting task. Some factors that will significantly impact needs have not yet emerged. Conversely, some factors that have been forecast may turn out differently than predicted. These unknown dynamics will influence the number and type of physicians needed in Alaska. Given the limitations of all predictions, the Task Force advises that the strategies recommended for achieving an adequate physician supply in Alaska be reviewed and updated regularly to insure that they are guided by current information.

B. Goals and Strategy Recommendations

Four goals encompass the strategies needed to address the physician supply in Alaska over the next 25 years.

Goals:

1. Increase the in-state production of physicians by increasing the number and viability of medical school and residency positions in Alaska and for Alaskans.

2. Increase the recruitment of physicians to Alaska by assessing needs and coordinating recruitment efforts.

3. Expand and support programs that prepare Alaskans for medical careers.

4. Increase retention of physicians by improving the practice environment in Alaska.

These goals and the related strategies are summarized below. Short-term strategies are those that require less than 5 years to impact the physician supply, medium-term strategies require 5–20 years and long-term strategies are expected to have an effect in more than 20 years. In the subsequent sections, each strategy is discussed in depth, including an explanation of the problem, related action steps, timeframe, benefit, cost, responsible party(ies), impact, and rationale. Further discussion including a review of the literature is included for each strategy.

Goals and Strategies for Securing an Adequate Physician Supply for Alaska's Needs

Major goal	Strategy	Timeline for impact	Estimated cost
1. Increase the in-state production of physicians by increasing the number and viability of medical school and residency positions in Alaska and for Alaskans.	A. Increase the number of state-subsidized medical school positions (WWAMI) from 10 to 30 per year.	Medium	$250,000 per practicing physician.
	B. Ensure financial viability of the AFMR through State support including Medicaid support.	Short	$60,000 per practicing physician.
	C. Increase the number of residency positions in Alaska, both in family medicine and appropriate additional specialties.	Short	$100,000 per year plus $30,000 for planning in year 1 & 2.

Goals and Strategies for Securing an Adequate Physician Supply for Alaska's Needs—Continued

Major goal	Strategy	Timeline for impact	Estimated cost
	D. Assist Alaskan students to attend medical school by: (i) reactivating and funding the use of the WICHE with a service obligation attached, and (ii) evaluating the possibility of seats for Alaskans in the planned osteopathic school at the Pacific Northwest University of the Health Science.	Medium	(i) $550,000 per practicing physician for WICHE; (ii) cost unknown at time of PSTF report.
	E. Investigate mechanisms for increasing Alaska-based experiences and education for WWAMI Students.	Medium	Unknown at time of PSTF Report.
	F. Maximize Medicare payments to teaching hospitals in Alaska.	Short	Zero cost to the State.
	G. Empanel a group to assess medical education in Alaska, including the viability of establishing an Alaska-based medical school.	Long	Undetermined at time of PSTF Report.
2. Increase the recruitment of physicians to Alaska by assessing needs and coordinating recruitment efforts.	A. Create a Medical Provider Workforce Assessment Office to monitor physician supply and facilitate physician recruitment efforts.	Short	$250,000 per year.
	B. Research and test a physician relocation incentive payment program.	Short	$65,000 per physician.
	C. Expand loan repayment assistance programs and funding for physicians practicing in Alaska.	Short	Undetermined—need to consult with other States.
3. Expand and support programs that prepare Alaskans for medical careers.	A. Expand and coordinate programs that prepare Alaskans for careers in medicine.	Medium	Up to $1,000,000 per year.
4. Increase retention of physicians by improving the practice environment in Alaska.	A. Develop a physician practice environment index for Alaska.	Short	$100,000 to develop index; $20,000 annually to update.
	B. Develop tools that promote community-based approaches to physician recruitment and retention.	Short	$50,000 per year.
	C. Support Federal tax credit legislation Initiative for physicians that meet frontier practice requirements.	Short	Zero cost to the State.

Goal 1. Increase the in-state production of physicians by increasing the number and viability of medical school and residency positions in Alaska and for Alaskans.

Strategy 1A. Increase the number of state-subsidized medical school positions (WWAMI) from 10 to 30 per year.

Problem. Alaska currently ranks 46th among U.S. States in terms of the number of state-supported medical school positions. Alaska ranks 49th among U.S. States in terms of the success of its applicants to U.S. medical schools, despite applicant qualifications equal to or better than the national average. Long-range planning, even if it includes a 4-year medical school in Alaska, will not address current physician needs in a timely fashion, so interim measures are needed.

Action Steps

1. WWAMI—Increase WWAMI positions to 20 per year and then potentially to 30 per year over a period of several years.

2. WICHE—Fund 10 additional seats per year via WICHE. Such funding should include a payback provision.

3. Monitor the rate of return and cost to benefit ratio.

4. Adjust the number of program seats available to reflect program objectives and outcomes, and to maximize accrual of physicians to Alaska from these programs.

Timeframe. Medium Term

Benefit. An increase of WWAMI positions by 10 per year will result in five additional physicians for Alaska each year. Providing 10 WICHE positions per year will result in two additional physicians for Alaska each year. Building in-state capacity for medical education supports long-term actions that will help to make Alaska more self-sufficient and less susceptible to outside factors that could negatively impact the health of Alaskans.

Cost. $400,000 per physician practicing in Alaska trained through WWAMI ($200,000/0.50); $600,000 per physician practicing in Alaska trained through WICHE ($110,000/0.18).

Responsibility. University of Washington, University of Alaska, Alaska State Legislature.

Impact. Training; Recruitment.

Rationale. A major determinant of the eventual practice location of physicians is where they went to medical school; so educating Alaskans in Alaska is likely to produce physicians for the State (COGME, 1998). Fifty percent of Alaskans who enter WWAMI practice in Alaska. Rate of return data for the Alaska WICHE physician programs suggest that 18 percent return to practice in the State.

Further Discussion. Increasing the number of WWAMI seats to 30 students would require a significant increase in resources at UAA to add capacity to serve the additional students. UAA would need to design and build additional facilities and to significantly increase the number of faculty in the program. It is difficult to accurately predict the amount of funding needed for the expansion. It has been suggested that enrollment be doubled to 20 in the medium term with the allocation of adequate funding, then re-examine the possibility of increasing to 30.

The cost to the State of a medical school position through WWAMI would be about $50,000 per student per year, or about $200,000 for the 4-year education of one student. With a 50 percent rate of return, each practicing Alaska physician costs $400,000. Increasing the class size from 10 to 20 students increases the total cost from about $2,000,000 to $4,000,000 per year. An additional increase to 30 students will add another $2,000,000 per year to the total.

Alaska can increase the number of state-subsidized medical school positions to 30 per year by either immediately increasing WWAMI positions to 20 per year and then building to 30 over a period of several years, and/or funding 10 additional seats per year via WICHE (with a payback provision). Over a period of several years these additional seats may be converted to WWAMI seats, depending on rate-of-return data.

WWAMI educates Alaskans in the State for as many as 3 of the 4 years of medical school. The program is recognized as one of the best medical school education programs in the country, especially for rural and primary care. Alaska's membership in the WICHE PSEP could be utilized to revise and re-establish the student loan program with a service obligation. Providing 10 WICHE positions per year will result in two additional physicians for Alaska each year. A payback provision may increase the number, but so many States now offer to pay off physician debt as a recruiting tool, the effect may not be large.

Since its inception in 1971, 50 percent of WWAMI graduates have returned to practice in Alaska. That percentage increases to 75 percent when WWAMI graduates from other WWAMI States are counted as "returned" WWAMI physicians. None of the graduates to date have been subject to the payback clause instituted in 1999, because it takes a minimum of 7 years before medical students are qualified for independent practice. Thus, the percentage returning to practice in Alaska may increase as those affected by the clause begin to enter practice, starting this year.

The Alaska Legislature has taken the first step in implementing this recommendation by appropriating $475,000 toward the one-time costs of doubling the WWAMI class size. This perceptive appropriation, anticipating an important State need, represents half of the required one-time costs and is an important first step to increase physician supply.

Under the WICHE program Alaskans can select from a variety of medical schools in western States. They apply independently and must be accepted in order to be eligible for their tuition to be subsidized by the State. The cost to the State of a medical school position through WICHE is about $26,000 per student per year ($25,600 for 2006–07, $26,500 projected for 2007–08 and $27,400 projected for 2008–09). Thus, the annual cost for 10 WICHE students in each of the 4-year medical school curriculum would be about $1,100,000. With an 18 percent rate of return, each practicing Alaska physician costs $610,000.

Increasing state-subsidized medical positions is a medium-term action that will provide a long-range payoff. Thus, it is part of an overall strategy to increase the number of physicians practicing in Alaska. However, it is an interim measure that is required until Alaska develops an in-state 4-year medical school.

"We need to 'grow our own.' Physicians tend to practice in the geographic area where they have completed their training or go back to where they have family. These factors mean that we need to expand both the Family Medicine Residency in Anchorage and the number of positions we have in WWAMI. "
—PETER MARSHALL, MD. PRIVATE PRACTICE, NORTH POLE,
CHAIRMAN, ALASKA WWAMI ADMISSIONS COMMITTEE.

Strategy 1B. Ensure financial viability of Alaska Family Medicine Residency through State support, including Medicaid support.

Problem. The AFMR operates at an annual loss of over $2,000,000. The sponsoring institution, Providence Alaska Medical Center, has been funding the deficit since the program's inception in 1997. The program's quality and viability are jeopardized by this dependence on private support, which could be withdrawn. Without such ongoing support the program would be forced to close, ending the only in-state GME program in Alaska.

Action Steps.

1. Work with State legislature to maximize Medicaid support of the AFMR.

2. Work with multiple State partners to revise Medicare policies that currently disfavor States with younger populations, such as Alaska.

3. Investigate ways to maximize Medicaid support for developing other GME programs in Alaska.

Timeframe. Short

Benefit. Directly places eight to nine family physicians per year in Alaska, a rate of placement that needs to be maintained.

Cost. $60,000 State cost per practicing physician. There would also be a cost for staff time to investigate additional Medicaid support of GME.

Responsible Entity. Alaska State Legislature with support of Alaska State Hospital and Nursing Association, Alaska State Medical Association, Department of Health and Social Services.

Impact. Training; Recruitment; Retention

Rationale. Seventy percent of AFMR's graduates remain in Alaska to practice. With 70 percent placed in Alaska, this gives Alaska the highest rate of return for GME in the United States (AAMC, 2006). Residency programs are one of the best ways to increase the number of physicians in a State (COGME, 1998). The AFMR is Alaska's only GME program, training 12 physicians per year. All States support their residency programs through a variety of funding mechanisms, including direct appropriation of funds. Currently Alaska has not maximized the amount of support for GME allowed under Federal law. By increasing the funding through Medicaid, Alaska would take advantage of the Federal Medicaid match, reducing the total State funds necessary. It is estimated that the AFMR is eligible for approximately $800,000 in additional Medicaid funds, under Federal law, which would require only an additional $400,000 of State appropriations.

Working with the State's Federal congressional delegation, changes in Medicare regulations can result in an additional payment of approximately $900,000 for the costs of rural training of residents in the program. Combined with increased Medicaid payments, this total of $1,700,000 brings the required program subsidy within $400,000. Other strategies to eliminate this deficit could include direct State appropriations, or further increases in the Medicaid payment rates for physician services (both are strategies used by other States). The final effect of achieving full funding will be to eliminate the program's financial vulnerability to cessation of private support.

Further Discussion. The AFMR is Alaska's only GME program. The program recruits and trains 12 doctors each year from Alaska and the United States. These doctors undergo a rigorous internship and residency program for 3 years, to become family physicians. The training emphasizes practice in rural and bush communities in Alaska and is very successful, placing over 70 percent of graduates in Alaska, over 50 percent in rural areas, and over 30 percent in tribal health practices, a performance achieved by very few, if any, other programs.

The total budget for the AFMR program is about $7,000,000 per year. The program operates at a deficit of over $2,000,000 per year. This is because the Medicare program, which funds most of GME nationwide, disfavors a young population like Alaska's. Consequently the sponsoring institution, Providence, receives only about half the reimbursement from Medicare that a similar hospital in the lower 48 would receive.

Other States support their family medicine residency programs with a combination of direct State appropriations, Medicaid payments for GME to hospitals, and increased Medicaid payment rates for the physician services provided by the residents and faculty. Alaska's Medicaid program provides $875,000 per year in support of the residency costs to Providence, and pays the regular physician rate for professional services to Medicaid patients. This rate is above the minimum rate Medicaid is required to pay for resident services, but not above the rate paid to non-academic physicians in private practice. There is no direct State appropriation.

Action by Alaska's congressional delegation may result in additional Federal support for the program totaling $800,000 per year, reducing the deficit to $1,200,000 annually. State support will be required to make up this deficit, to ensure the ongoing presence of the residency program.

Following trends in other States, Alaska has three obvious opportunities to secure the funding of the AFMR:

• increasing Medicaid GME funds to the sponsoring hospital to the maximum allowable will provide the program with $800,000, at a cost to the State of only $400,000;

• further increasing the payment rates for residency services to patients to the comparable private insurance payment rate is also allowable, and would provide the program an additional estimated $150,000 per year. (This would cost the State $75,000, due to the Federal matching benefits); and

• a direct State appropriation to support GME of $250,000 per year (very similar to support provided by other States).

Assuming the congressional efforts are successful, the State can ensure the viability of the AFMR by adopting these three measures. These measures will also create the environment where additional growth of residency programs and positions is possible in Alaska.

Funding needs breakdown:

Funding source	Amount	Deficit
Current funding	$7,000,000	$2,000,000
Medicare rule changes	800,000	1,200,000
Maximize Medicaid for GME	800,000	400,000
Maximize Medicaid fees	150,000	250,000
Direct State support	250,000	0

The supply of rural physicians depends largely on the production of family physicians. Although many factors contribute to the choice to practice in rural areas—rural upbringing, medical school attended, and special educational service experiences—the final common pathway for the largest number of rural physicians is a family medicine residency (Council on Graduate Medical Education, 1998). Some of the residents are recruited from the State's population, after they graduate from medical school. Typically, however, a majority of the residents are recruited from other medical schools, bringing new doctors into the State. Doctors, especially in family medicine, tend to stay and practice in the State where they finish their residencies, the last stage of training. All States in the United States have residency programs. Alaska was the last State to start a residency, and since Alaska has far fewer physicians per population than any other State in the Western United States, it is very important to keep a residency viable.

"I am from Fairbanks, Alaska. I chose the Alaska Family Practice residency primarily because it was in Alaska, where I wanted to be. It also helped that it was gaining a reputation for being an excellent residency."
—LEIF THOMPSON, MD. BRISTOL BAY AREA HEALTH CORPORATION.

One of the major obstacles to expanding GME in Alaska is the lack of funding. All the GME expansion strategies are unlikely to succeed if they cannot be operated at a "break even" level for the sponsoring institutions. The existing AFMR operates at a deficit, which jeopardizes its long-term viability. All States support their GME programs. By maximizing the use of Medicaid, the State leverages its investment through the Federal matching funds, thereby minimizing the cost to the State and maximizing support for the programs.

Alaska has not yet investigated thoroughly the ways to maximize Medicaid support for GME. Doing so would require staff time to research the issue and discuss with colleagues in other States. Most of the necessary changes can be done administratively within Alaska's Medicaid program. Within a year, new GME funds could be made available, provided the analysis reveals opportunity. Once funds are available, hospitals statewide will be in a position to explore starting GME programs.

Strategy 1C. Increase number of residency positions in Alaska, both in family medicine and appropriate additional specialties.

Problem. Currently Alaska ranks last among west coast States in the number of medical residents in training per capita. Limited number of residency training opportunities contributes to the statewide physician shortage.

Action Steps. Increase the number of residency positions in Alaska by the following mechanisms.

1. Increase the number of short-term resident rotations in Alaska by coordination and marketing.

2. Develop "Alaska Tracks" in collaboration with established residencies in other States to provide significant parts of training in Alaska.

3. Develop additional full-fledged residencies in Alaska, as conditions permit.

4. Establish a central agency to coordinate, track and develop additional residency experiences.

Timeframe. Short term. Two to six years.

Benefit. Residencies in Alaska or sponsored for Alaskans in other States impact the number of physicians who choose to practice in Alaska. Increasing the number of residency options and implementing an "Alaska Tracks" program would result in net gains to Alaska's physician supply each year.

Cost. $100,000 per year. "Alaska Tracks" could gain funding from Medicare, if located in rural areas under certain conditions that need to be explored to determine feasibility. This funding could cover half or more of the cost of the programs. The State portion would depend on the number and length of the programs.

Planning for additional residencies would cost approximately $30,000 per year for 1 to 2 years. Operational costs for new residencies would depend greatly on the size, location and specialty. The current budget for the AFMR is over $7,000,000 per year.

Responsibility. For appropriations, Alaska State Legislature. For operations, AFMR.

Impact. Training; Recruitment.

Rationale. Local resident training is a very effective way of increasing doctors in a State. Up to 70 percent of residents ultimately enter practice in the State where they train (Council on Graduate Medical Education, 1998). Since residencies are major determinants of practice location of physicians, it is important that Alaska maximize its opportunities to offer residency positions in State. Alaska could offer residency tracks as an adjunct to programs in other States, and/or Alaska could be more efficient in supporting residencies for Alaskans completing residencies in other States.

Further Discussion. Currently, Alaska can maximize the number of short-term, 1- to 2-month rural experiences associated with residencies in other States. A number of these are coordinated by DHSS (NHSC SEARCH: Alaskan Exposure program) and ANTHC's tribal sites. Many of these experiences are currently arranged based on the interest of the resident and availability of sites. There is some coordination across these programs but no mechanism exists for centralized coordination. A central coordinating agency should be established to coordinate, track and develop these experiences.

Opportunities for increasing the number of resident rotations in Alaska may exist in psychiatry in Juneau, in surgery in Fairbanks, in a variety of specialties in Anchorage and the Mat-Su Valley, and in many Alaska Native tribal health care system hospitals in rural areas. Residents frequently seek opportunities in Alaska, and a better system of marketing and coordination could increase the number of residents coming to the State.

Development of additional full residencies in Alaska may be difficult, but adding "Alaska Tracks" as part of existing residencies in other States may be more feasible. Currently, the Alaska Native Medical Center (ANMC) has a 3-to-6-month track for surgical residents from a program in Arizona; all the practicing surgeons at ANMC came from this program. Fairbanks Memorial Hospital is working to develop a similar program with the University of Washington. In Boise, the VA hospital has a 1-year (of three total) track for internists from the UW. Such tracks are much more effective in recruiting doctors than short 1 or 2 month rotations, but less effective than a full residency program. "Alaska Tracks" could be available in many specialties in many parts of the State. There are many barriers to this approach, most importantly the ability and willingness of residencies in other States to send their trainees to Alaska. There may be significant loss of funding to the home programs when residents leave.

The feasibility of establishing residencies in Alaska in addition to the AFMR should be carefully and critically evaluated. Current Medicare law does not allow new residencies to be funded, except in rural areas. However, rural parts of the State lack the physician specialists and patient types and volumes to support residencies in most specialties. Even in Anchorage the same issues limit the possible programs to pediatrics, internal medicine, psychiatry, and perhaps a few others. But, again, Medicare funding would not be available. The AHEC and the AFMR should study this option and work with existing institutions to develop plans for implementation.

Additional 1-to-2-month rural rotations would have a net recruitment rate of 10–15 percent. Assuming as many as 30 additional rotations would become available; this would net Alaska an additional three to five doctors per year. These recruits would begin practicing as soon as 2 years after the program started.

The recruitment rate from "Alaska Tracks" would be higher, probably in the 20–30 percent range, depending on the specialty and the length of the track. A longer track would have a higher recruitment rate, but could accommodate fewer doctors per year. If three different tracks were developed, exposing 10 residents per year, the net would be two to three doctors, starting 2 years after inception.

The AHEC could prepare a report on the feasibility of new residencies in 1 to 2 years. If a new program were planned, a minimum of 2 years would be required to develop it, achieve accreditation and start training. The production of the program would begin 3 to 4 years later. The output would be four to six doctors per year, of whom three to five would remain in State, beginning in 2012.

"Alaska Tracks" could gain funding from Medicare, if located in rural areas and not in Alaska Native tribal health care system hospitals. This funding could cover half or more of the cost of the programs. The State portion would depend on the number and length of the programs.

A professional estimate is that planning for additional residencies would cost approximately $30,000 per year for 1 to 2 years. Actually operating a residency would depend greatly on the size and location and specialty. The current budget for the AFMR is over $7,000,000 per year.

The supply of rural physicians is largely dependent on the production of family physicians. Although many factors contribute to the choice to practice in rural areas, including rural upbringing, medical school attended, and special educational service experiences. The final common pathway for the largest number of rural physicians is a family medicine residency (Council on Graduate Medical Education, 1998. p. 23).

Strategy 1D. Assist Alaskan students to attend medical school by: (i) reactivating and funding the use of WICHE PSEP with a service obligation attached, and (ii) evaluating the possibility of seats for Alaskans in the planned osteopathic school at the Pacific Northwest University of the Health Sciences.

Problem. Alaska lacks adequate state-funded financial supports for Alaskan students in medical school, and the State lacks state-subsidized positions at an osteopathic school.

Action Steps.

1. Utilize Alaska's membership in the WICHE Professional Student Exchange Program to revise and re-establish the student loan program with a service obligation.

2. Explore the possibility with the Pacific Northwest University of Health Sciences, in Yakima, Washington of seats for Alaskans in the new osteopathic school upon its completion, which is scheduled for Fall, 2008.

Timeframe. Mid term. Five to ten years.

Benefit. This strategy helps State residents afford medical education while simultaneously providing the state/community with a quantifiable pool of future medical professionals. Loan repayment and other direct financial incentives have the benefit of insuring that any funds expended are associated with an individual practitioner providing a service. Alaskan student slots in the osteopathic school would boost the number of Alaskans attending medical school and impact the number of physicians who choose to practice in the State.

Cost. The cost of the WICHE PSEP action step is projected to be $550,000 per practicing physician. The cost of guaranteed slots in the osteopathic school in Yakima is unknown at time of this report.

Responsible Entities. For Federal appropriations, Alaska Congressional Delegation. For appropriation of operational funds, Alaska State Legislature.

An operational entity, such as a board or task force, needs to be established that can set policy regarding the level of subsidies, the manner in which the subsidies are to be deployed, and other financial strategies to best meet health care workforce needs. The proposed Medical Provider Workforce Assessment Office would investigate these strategies and provide information to the entity making the policy decisions. The Alaska Commission on Postsecondary Education would be the most likely organization to administer the financial support programs. For the medical school seats, discussions would be needed with Pacific Northwest University of the Health Sciences.

Impact. Training; Recruitment; Retention.

Rationale. Loan repayment, direct incentive, and loan programs have been found to be effective for recruitment and retention (Pathman, et al., 2004). Past WICHE students with service requirements account for a number of physicians who have stayed in Alaska after the service pay-back that was required previously. However, State funds were cut to the WICHE program in 1995. The Task Force determined that the State student aid program with a service obligation should be funded again by the State. Additionally, educating Alaskans with seats at the DO school is likely to build the pipeline and produce physicians for the State.

Further Discussion. The WICHE PSEP provided loans to medical students in participating schools, with an obligation to return to the State to practice, but Alaska has not participated in the medical school component for 10 years.

Increases in financial supports for medical education are needed to build the number of Alaskans in the physician supply pipeline, and to strengthen recruitment and retention strategies. Through their deliberations, the members of the Physician Supply Task Force considered the five recognized types of incentives to encourage physicians to practice in underserved areas: scholarships, service-option loans, loan repayment, direct financial incentives, and resident support.

Loan repayment and other direct financial incentives have the benefit of insuring that any funds expended are associated with an individual practitioner providing a service (in contrast to the contingent loans, which must be administered for either the life of the service commitment or for the entire repayment period). Additionally, the benefit can be made available to draw residents of other States to Alaska. These options would also have relatively low administrative costs.

A national study assessed all State programs that provided financial support to medical students, residents and practicing physicians in exchange for a period of service in underserved areas. Compared to young non-obligated physicians, physicians serving obligations to State programs were more satisfied and remained in their practices longer, half of them staying over 8 years. Retention rates were highest for loan repayment, direct incentive, and loan programs. These State programs target physicians at the end of their training, when they know more about their career interests, job options, and family needs (Pathman, et al., 2004).

The current PSEP support fees for each medical student beginning their GME in 2007 would be a total of $111,400 over 4 years. The cost of loan repayment/direct financial incentives currently is undetermined. Alaska would need to identify what other States are doing and figure out what a reasonable "tipping point" is to insure the repayment cap is high enough and/or financial incentive substantial enough to be effective.

Strategy 1E. Investigate mechanisms for increasing Alaska-based experiences and education for WWAMI students.

Problem. Currently, medical students in Alaska's sole medical education program, WWAMI, complete their first year in Anchorage. They have the option to complete nearly all of the third year and large parts of the fourth year in Alaska. Second year classes for all WWAMI students are held in Seattle.

Action Step. Work with University of Washington WWAMI, the University of Alaska and the Alaska medical profession to investigate the feasibility and cost of providing all WWAMI first and second year classes and third and fourth year clerkships in Alaska.

Timeframe. Medium term.

Benefit. Providing rotations in all 4 years of medical school in Alaska will make the State more independent, able to negotiate economies of scale and more independent in setting class size according to State needs.

Cost. Undetermined at time of Task Force Report. Responsibility. University of Alaska, University of Washington Impact. Training; Recruitment.

Rationale. Medical students who experience increased exposure to Alaska through in-state training, rotations, clerkships and other experiences in Alaska are more likely to practice in the State (COGME, 2004).

"We need to offer more support for the Alaska students who attend medical school in other States. They should be considered part of our 'family'. They should be offered some type of financial deal and/or electives in Alaska that may

encourage them to return to the State to practice. The physicians in Fairbanks and Fairbanks Memorial Hospital have purchased diagnostic kits to give to the students who are accepted into the WWAMI Program. We also have a few kits that we will be awarding to some of the students who are going to medical school elsewhere."

—PETER MARSHALL, MD. PRIVATE PRACTICE, NORTH POLE,
CHAIRMAN, ALASKA WWAMI ADMISSIONS COMMITTEE.

Strategy IF. Maximize Medicare payments to teaching hospitals in Alaska.

Problem. Current levels of Medicare support for GME in Alaska are inadequate to cover teaching hospital expenses. The current payment formulas are biased against States with young populations such as Alaska, because the formulas are driven by the number of Medicare patients in the teaching hospital. Alaska-based GME is jeopardized by this funding deficit.

Action Steps.

1. Continue to maximize existing opportunities for Medicare coverage for GME.
2. Identify and advocate for specific areas where additional Medicare coverage would be beneficial to GME in Alaska.

Timeframe. Short term. Within 5 years.

Benefits. Changes to Medicare payment formulas to reflect GME expenses would stabilize GME programs in States with younger populations by providing a long-term funding stream. These changes will need to be led by the Federal delegation.

Cost. Zero cost to the State, as this is a Federal funding stream. The total Federal cost would depend on the formula changes and the number of programs that subsequently develop.

Responsibility. Alaska Federal Congressional Delegation supported by Alaska State Medical Association, Alaska State Hospital and Nursing Association, statewide health care partners.

Impact. Training; Recruitment.

Rationale. Medicare is the primary funder of GME nationwide. Establishing new formulas specific to rural or frontier States would allow a more even distribution of Medicare funds. Changes in Medicare statutes/regulations are needed to help stabilize GME in Alaska.

Further Discussion. Current levels of Federal support for GME in Alaska are inadequate. The Federal laws establishing and regulating GME payments through the Medicare program are designed to provide marginally adequate funding for large teaching hospitals on the east coast. The number of Medicare patients in the teaching hospital drives the formulas. Alaska, having a young population, has a much smaller proportion of Medicare patients than other States. The funding that is marginal in New York is completely inadequate in Alaska. Improving the payment rates for Alaska will require new formulas specific to rural or frontier States, and/or alteration in Medicare regulations. These changes will need to be led by the Federal delegation.

If it becomes possible to alter Federal law, programs would develop in the State alone or in concert with GME programs from other States. Alteration of the formulas to more evenly distribute the funds would give Alaska a long-term recurring stream of funds.

Strategy 1G. Empanel a group to assess medical education in Alaska, including the viability of establishing an Alaska-based medical school.

Problem. Alaska does not have an independent 4-year medical school nor does it have a sufficient number of slots in other State programs for qualified Alaskans to pursue medical education. This deficit in training capacity contributes to the shortage of physicians in Alaska. Currently, no entity exists to explore options and strategically plan for medical education in Alaska. There is no strategic plan for medical education in Alaska that allows for rational reassessment and planning to accommodate continually changing State needs.

Action Step. Empanel a group or charge an existing group to develop a strategic plan for medical education in Alaska that will define the requirements (including cost estimates) and the potential benefits (including economic impact) of a 4-year medical school in Alaska and ensure continued adherence to this recommendation as needs change.

Timeframe. Long term.

Benefit. This recommendation develops options for the State of Alaska. A rational strategic planning process will ensure that medical education in Alaska will develop in a way that will maximize the State's return on its investment, producing the largest number of physicians, as needed. A 4-year medical school in the State would provide significant economic benefit and an enhanced practice environment to encourage physician recruitment, and would provide increased opportunity to develop one of Alaska's most precious resources, young Alaskans seeking professional medical education.

If continuing collaborative medical education with other WWAMI participants is in the State's best interest, that partnership can be maintained. If a more independent medical school is more appropriate, then the program is positioned to take that next sequential step.

Based on the current number of medical school applications by Alaskans, their qualifications and reasonable projections, implementing this strategy could provide 30 physicians per year by 2020, about 23 more than the current WWAMI program.

Cost. Undetermined at time of Task Force Report.

Responsibility. New empanelled group to investigate State medical education.

Impact. Training; Recruitment.

Rationale. Alaska lacks the benefits enjoyed by States with 4-year medical schools. These benefits include: a significant boost to regional economy, stimulation of associated businesses, a more attractive recruiting environment for physicians, an improved medical practice environment, and better health status in the State. A rational strategic plan is needed to insure that Alaska has an adequate physician supply through 2025. The creation of an Alaska medical school would allow more of the State's resources to remain in the State, developing capacity and infrastructure in Alaska.

Further Discussion. Rational planning for medical education requires that there be regular, critical evaluation of the potential for future development. This task should be charged to an appropriate planning group. The alternative is a crisis management approach that often leads to sudden, wholesale changes that challenge the maintenance of a quality educational program.

While medical education in Alaska has the greatest potential to supply future Alaskan physicians, the current class size in WWAMI relegates it to a miniscule role in physician supply. Currently, class size cannot be changed easily. Agreement is needed by the University of Alaska Anchorage, the University of Washington School of Medicine, statewide offices of the University of Alaska and the Alaska Legislature to change the class size. Alaska currently participates in a very successful medical education program, WWAMI, but there are minimal economies of scale as class size increases.

There is little doubt that Alaska will have a medical school in the future. There are many examples of small States with their own medical schools, including States with far less resources. Until that time, Alaska should work to nurture and develop its current medical education program (WWAMI) in ways that support the development of a more complete in-state program, or a freestanding medical school. Sequential development within the existing medical education program will maintain the high quality of the program currently in place.

Implementing these provisions could provide 30 physicians per year by 2020, about 23 more than the current program. This number assumes a medical school class of about 50, selected from an anticipated applicant pool of more than 100 applicants. There are between 70 and 80 Alaska applicants per year. About half of all applicants are qualified for admission. Other applicants could be drawn from outside Alaska.

The medical education program in Alaska can be responsive to changing State needs by readily accommodating changes in the number of students admitted and allowing economies of scale to be realized when class size increases.

Goal 2. Increase the recruitment of physicians to Alaska by assessing needs and coordinating recruitment efforts.

Strategy 2A. Create a medical provider workforce assessment office to monitor physician supply and facilitate physician recruitment efforts

Problem. Currently there is no statewide entity with sufficient resources to adequately coordinate and address medical provider workforce issues. Effective planning for future physician supply is hindered because there is no office with an ongoing responsibility to regularly assess physician supply and need, and research and report on medical provider data. Alaska's medical provider recruitment efforts are disjointed, resulting in higher recruitment costs and duplicate efforts by various organizations.

Action Steps.

1. Establish a centralized, statewide Medical Provider Workforce Assessment Office.

2. Develop performance standards and measures for the Medical Provider Workforce Assessment Office.

3. Implement scope of work and tasks of the Medical Provider Workforce Assessment Office.

Timeframe. Short term. 12-18 months.

Benefit. A Medical Provider Workforce Assessment Office would result in ongoing assessment of the status of medical provider supply, support long-term planning efforts, directly contribute to net gains in physician supply, and improve the cost efficiency of Alaska's medical provider workforce recruitment.

Cost estimate. $250,000 per year. Costs should be shared between the organizations concerned with physician and other medical provider workforce and the State of Alaska. The office could establish fees for its services in addition to this core appropriation.

Responsibility. The Medical Provider Workforce Assessment Office should be located in the State of Alaska, Department of Health and Social Services.

Impact. Recruitment; Retention

Rationale. Assuring access to health care is a State public health function. A key component of access to health care is an adequate medical workforce. Assessment of the status of the health care workforce, including physicians, and the impact on health status is a critical activity and warrants a focused and coordinated response by a Medical Provider Workforce Assessment Office.

As well as assessing and reporting the adequacy of the medical provider workforce, the Medical Provider Workforce Assessment Office would play a critical role in responding to provider shortages by facilitating and marketing recruiting activities statewide among all potential employers and practices in the State.

Further Discussion. The two primary areas of focus for the proposed Medical Provider Workforce Assessment Office include the study and analysis of the medical provider workforce, including physicians; and the facilitation and support of recruitment activities.

Alaska needs a centralized office in order to identify and track physician supply, trends, and practice. The Alaska Physician Supply Task Force report is the first report to determine the supply and need for physicians and to identify action steps to affect the supply. Ongoing assessment is needed of the multiple data sets from national, State, regional and local sources that were used by the Task Force.

Other States have created an office similar to the proposed Medical Provider Workforce Assessment Office, with good results. The envisioned program would be run from a State office, most likely from the Department of Health and Social Services. A precedent for such an office is the Alaska Seafood Marketing Institute. The Medical Provider Workforce Assessment Office would document the status of the medical provider workforce, assess the market, and work with multiple stakeholders to plan a recruitment strategy that would assist where needed and avoid interference where appropriate.

The Medical Provider Workforce Assessment Office would share information about physician supply and recruitment "best practices" across sites to help minimize costs and reduce duplication in recruitment efforts and to promote ongoing policy discussions regarding physician availability. The Task Force recognized that hospitals and other entities will want to continue their own specific recruitment activities.

Workforce development activities exist in multiple locations including the tribally managed system, private sector, and various State and Federal agencies. However existing programs are not monitoring or analyzing specialty distribution or needs, changing roles of mid-level providers, or potential impact of electronic health records on all providers. Coordination of the efforts, and research and analysis of relevant trends, should inform policy.

Strategy 2B. Research and test a physician re-location incentive pay program.

Problem. The ability to attract and retain physicians to care for medically underserved populations is compromised due to the high expense of establishing a practice in Alaska as compared to other States.

Action Steps.

1. Research relocation incentive pay programs in other States.
2. Research Federal laws related to provision of relocation incentive pay.
3. Design and implement a relocation incentive pay pilot program.

Timeframe. Short term. Six to twelve months.

Benefit. If successful, this strategy would give Alaska another method to attract physicians to medically underserved areas. It would contribute to a more favorable practice climate resulting in a net gain of physicians willing to provide care for medically underserved populations.

Cost. Estimated cost of $65,000 one-time funds to secure one physician. This includes approximately $15,000 for travel related expenses plus up to $50,000 for a financial incentive payment depending on specialty of physician selected. Research and design efforts would be funded through the proposed Medical Provider Workforce Assessment Office (Strategy 2A).

Responsibility. ASMA, Alaska State Hospital and Nursing Association, proposed Medical Provider Workforce Assessment Office.

Impact. Recruitment; Retention.

Rationale. Many States have established programs that offer a signing bonus to compete effectively for the limited number of physicians, especially in medically underserved areas. This pilot program would provide an opportunity to determine the efficacy of a relocation bonus in securing physicians for medically underserved populations in Alaska. This strategy and related action steps will need to address requirements of Stark regulations that prohibit hospitals from providing direct financial incentives to physicians.

Further Discussion. There are challenges in attracting physicians to Alaska to establish a practice, or to remain in practice if already in the State. One of those is the expense of establishing a practice in Alaska compared to other States due to higher salaries, office expenses, and uncompensated care burden. Other factors include affordable housing, malpractice expense, cost to periodically visit family out of State, and generally higher family expenses at a time when many new physicians are burdened with medical school debt that must be repaid. Newly established physicians do not have the financial flexibility to cover all of these higher costs of living in Alaska, which may cause them to consider more economically advantageous locations around the United States.

Alaska must identify creative ways to reduce the financial gap between establishing a practice in Alaska versus other States. A number of States have created programs that offer a signing bonus to attract physicians in return for a set commitment in years to stay in that State.

Alaska should test the feasibility of a physician relocation incentive pilot program. The pilot program should be based on:

- a review of design and effectiveness of other States' programs, looking at overall return on investment for the bonuses awarded;
- the estimated amount of signing bonus needed to effectively impact a physician's decision to establish a practice in Alaska;
- the estimated cost to administer the program and most appropriate agency to house the responsibility;
- the scope of specialties that would be eligible for this program;
- areas of the State that would be given priority for award of these bonuses;
- initial discussions included rural and underserved communities that do not have the resources to offer these bonuses on their own;
- an analysis of Federal laws impact on this strategy, specifically the Federal Stark provisions;
- the estimated cost for administering a full scale program and number of placements that could be supported; and
- the amount of signing bonus needed to effectively impact a physician's decision.

Many States have a program that offers a signing bonus simply to compete effectively for the limited number of physicians looking to start or relocate their practice. These signing bonuses generally come with a 3- to 5-year practice commitment to avoid repayment of the bonus if the physician leaves the State early. This strategy would target already established physicians who wish to leave their current location as well as physicians completing a residency program and planning to establish their first practice. Members of the Alaska Legislative leadership did not support a request for funding a financial incentive program during the 2006 Session in part because they wanted evidence that this strategy would produce results. This pilot program would provide an opportunity to demonstrate whether Alaska could be successful competing with other States/organizations. If successful, this strategy could be presented as part of a comprehensive set of recommendations to the Alaska Legislature to create statutory authority and financing to fund a full-scale program to recruit physicians.

Alaskans for Access to Health Care (AAHC) has been actively involved in this Legislative session to bring attention to the need to invest funding to attract physicians to Alaska. AAHC is made up of ASHNHA, ASMA, Alaska Physicians and Surgeons, and Providence Alaska Health Systems. AAHC is informally referred to as "ACCESS." It would be helpful for ACCESS members and Alaska DHSS to continue exploring financing a pilot effort to travel to physician conferences, medical school campuses, large residency settings and other opportune locations to promote the benefits of an Alaska practice and to offer financial incentives to choose Alaska for their practice.

If successful, this strategy would give Alaska another effective selling point along with the other strategies in this document to attract physicians. Clearly this would not be the primary ingredient in each physician's decision when choosing a practice location, but it would perhaps tip the scale in enough cases to warrant funding a program of this type on a permanent basis.

Strategy 2C. Expand loan repayment assistance programs and funding for physicians practicing in Alaska.

Problem. The main loan repayment programs available to physicians in Alaska are provided through IHS and NSHC. Limitations of these programs are that funding is restricted and subject to annual cutbacks that threaten their stability, and that only certain practice locations and specialties are eligible for loan repayment through these programs.

In order to gain more physicians Alaska could participate in the HRSA Bureau of Health Professions (BHPr) State Loan Repayment Program which has a 50/50 State and Federal match, but Alaska is one of 13 States that do not participate. In addition, Alaska does not have its own SLRP for physicians committing to practice in Alaska in specialties or areas not allowed in the Federal programs (including the SLRP).

Action Steps.

1. Identify opportunities to apply for the HRSA Bureau of Health Professions SLRP and a supplemental State loan repayment program.

2. Work with DHSS, Governor, State Legislature, and/or local communities to secure the 50 percent State match required for the HRSA BHPr SLRP.

3. Research the structure of physician loan repayment programs in other States.

4. Fund a State loan repayment program to supplement the Federal loan repayment programs, for physicians serving in shortage areas designated by the State.

5. Identify and work with an agency to administer the HRSA BHPr SLRP and/or the supplemental State loan repayment program.

6. Continue informing Alaska's national delegates of the need to maintain or increase annual Federal allocations for NHSC loan repayment program and IHS loan repayment program.

Timeframe. Short term. One to two years.

Benefit. Improved Federal funding will enable the IHS and NHSC loan repayment programs to be stabilized and will allow more clinical sites to recruit physicians. This will support rural placements including tribal facilities and community health centers. Alaska's participation in the HRSA SLRP would allow more physicians in the general specialties to work in underserved areas. With an Alaska State loan repayment program not tied to HRSA BHPr, the State could more easily recruit not only general specialists but also other physician specialists that are needed and could use state-designated shortage areas so that many additional sites would be eligible.

Cost. Undetermined at time of Task Force Report.

With an Alaska State loan repayment program not tied to HRSA BHPr, the State could more easily recruit not only general specialists but other physician specialists that are needed, and many additional sites could be eligible for loan repayment.

Under the IHS loan repayment program, applicants sign contractual agreements for 2 years and fulfill their agreements through full-time clinical practice at an IHS facility or Alaskan Native tribal health program. In return, the LRP will repay all or a portion of the applicant's eligible health professional educational loans (undergraduate and graduate) for tuition expenses. Applicants are eligible to have their educational loans repaid in amounts up to $20,000 per year for each year of service, tax-free. Eligible specialties are family medicine, internal medicine, pediatrics, geriatric medicine, obstetrics and gynecology, and podiatric medicine. Currently there are 18 physicians working in Alaska with IHS loan repayment.

> *"Physicians carry a heavy burden of debt coming out of training and are attracted to areas where a healthy share of that burden can be taken away."*
> —JOHN BRINGHURST, CEO, PETERSBURG MEDICAL CENTER.

Goal 3. Expand and support programs that prepare Alaskans for medical careers.

Strategy 3A. Expand and coordinate programs that prepare Alaskans for careers in medicine.

Problem. Too few Alaskan high school students choose to pursue a career in medicine. Opportunities that would motivate a greater number of middle and high school students to pursue medicine as a career path are lost due to lack of medical career counseling, insufficient academic preparedness in math and science, and insufficient exposure to careers in medicine made available through school programs.

Alaska ranks 49th among U.S. States in terms of the success of its applicants to United States medical schools, despite applicant qualifications at, or better than, the national average.

Action Steps.

1. Expand and coordinate programs which prepare students for careers in medicine.

2. Provide financial support to effective programs that provide in school and summer experiences, internships and job shadowing.

3. Provide support to programs that make math and science available to K–12 students.

4. Facilitate clinical rotations to rural and underserved areas.

5. Provide State support for an industry/university partnership geared to encourage youth into health careers.

6. Support current programs to attract students to health careers.

7. Create a Web site and clearinghouse for opportunities and experiences in health careers.

8. Strengthen the Alaska AHEC by providing State support and by increasing number of regional AHEC centers required to accomplish above stated goals.

Timeframe. Medium term of 10–15 years for impact.

Benefits. The benefits of implementing this strategy and action steps are that students will be more academically prepared for medical school. The long-term benefit of this strategy will be an increased number of Alaskan students who select medicine as their career.

Cost. Provide up to $1,000,000 in State matching funds for Federal pipeline programs.

Responsibility. University of Alaska, Alaska AHEC, State of Alaska, Alaska State Legislature.

Impact. Training

Rationale. Alaska must grow its own pool of academic talent to prepare for careers in medical education. To support this growth and adequately prepare Alaskan students for a career in medicine, more attention needs to be directed to preparing and exposing students to related careers in a meaningful way within their community. Today there are too few opportunities to expose students to the realities and the excitement of these careers. The opportunities that do exist are not well known.

Further Discussion. Alaska has a variety of programs that address specific components of the health workforce and the training curriculum. Coordination between programs is sporadic at best, resulting in gaps and redundancies. A communication venue and tracking database, which facilitates coordination between and among the various Alaskan agencies supporting the development of Alaska's health workforce is needed.

Most programs supporting the health workforce curriculum do not receive sufficient funding to support long-term tracking, let alone the development of intermediate impact measures. This compromises their ability to advocate for future funding. An on-line database with a self-administering format and protected access reduces barriers to both tracking students and coordinating student participation across programs.

Based on interviews conducted across Alaska in 2004, and corroborated by national data, a primary reason for youth not to select careers in medicine is lack of exposure to those opportunities (Elder, 1997; Alexander, 2003; Bumgarner, 2003; Gill, 1996; Ramsey, 2001; Magzoub, 2000 and Weiler, 1997).

In Alaska, attrition and recruitment costs are the highest in remote, underserved regions (DHSS/ACRH, 2006). Research shows that tangible, positive clinical experience in a setting prior to graduation is a factor in encouraging graduates to select that setting for employment (Boulger, 2000; Jones, 2000; Neill, 2002; Ramsey, 2001; Bacon, 2000; and Rabinowitz, 1999).

It is important to provide regionally tailored activities with measurable outcomes to expose youth to information about careers in medicine and a tangible connection to those opportunities. These would include speaker's bureaus to high schools, summer immersion programs and job shadowing in local health facilities. Additionally, efforts must be made to reach out to all those who are currently applying to medical school to give them coaching for applications and interviews.

Goal 4. Increase retention of physicians by improving the practice environment in Alaska.

Strategy 4A. Develop a physician practice environment index for Alaska.

Problem. Alaska lacks an objective and reliable method to compare its physician practice environment to that in other States.

Action Step. Develop a practice environment assessment and comparison tool. Similar tools currently exist for other States and can be modified for Alaska.

Timeframe. Short term. Within 2 to 3 years.

Benefit. This strategy would provide an objective basis to measure Alaska's physician practice environment relative to other States and the national average. The index would identify elements that cause Alaska's practice environment to be relatively better or worse than other States. This would provide indications for strategies that could better the environment. Also, it would identify those elements that are strong, relative to other States, and therefore should be stressed in the recruiting process.

Cost. $100,000 to develop the physician practice environment index. $20,000 annually to update.

Responsibility. Medical Provider Workforce Assessment Office and health care partners.

Impact. Recruitment; Retention.

Rationale. The various elements that together constitute the practice environment need to be identified and quantified in a manner that allows comparison to the entire United States as well as to other States. It can serve as a mechanism that would suggest the specific element or elements that cause Alaska to rank either higher or lower. Such objective measures can provide the basis for strategies to strengthen or improve a particular element as well as an objective way to market the elements in which it has relatively higher strengths.

Further Discussion. An important part of the index would be the relative weightings among the various elements in the practice environment. For example, one expected element could be the medical-legal climate. One measure that could be used for this element would be physician professional liability premium rates. This element, for example, could receive a higher relative weighting. In a 2003 survey, 62 percent of medical residents stated that the most important aspect in practice environment was the medical liability environment (Merit, 2003).

At least one other State has developed such an index. The Massachusetts Medical Society (MMS) developed an index 5 years ago based on nine elements that are weighted based on their importance to the overall practice environment. The base year is 1992, and MMS has developed the index for each year from 1992 through 2005 for the United States and Massachusetts. It hires an economic consulting firm to do the statistical analysis. The MMS index could provide a starting point for developing an Alaskan Physician Practice Index.

Cost would probably depend on who will conduct the analysis given that template exists in Massachusetts and that the medical community could be tapped for volunteer, expert input, $100,000 would probably be sufficient funding for the initial development. Annual index development and re-calculation would probably not exceed $20,000 per year.

The Task Force identified the University of Alaska, Institute for Social and Economic Research as an organization that potentially could coordinate development and implementation of the index.

Strategy 4B. Develop tools that promote community-based approaches to physician recruitment and retention.

Problem. Practice sites and communities engaged in physician recruitment efforts are often less successful because they are unaware of factors that influence physician practice location and effective strategies to improve recruitment outcomes.

Action Steps.

1. Provide tools for technical assistance and training on physician shortage and the impact of site development efforts.

2. Provide tools to form community-based organizations, such as community health councils, to address local site development (U.S. DHHS, 2006).

3. Develop promotional materials that highlight community resources and economy as a component of the physician recruitment efforts (Commonwealth, 2005. p. 30).

4. Increase the partnerships among health care sites and organizations, such as Chambers of Commerce and Economic Development Councils that can help promote the community as a desirable practice location.

Timeframe. Short term. Twelve to eighteen months.

Benefits. This strategy would result in more appropriate matches between communities and physicians. As a result, physicians seeking employment would find Alaska practice sites and communities to be more desirable. The anticipated benefits are shorter length of vacancies, increased number of hires, and increased length of retention.

Cost. $50,000 per year.

Responsibility. Proposed Medical Provider Workforce Assessment Office and health care partners.

Impact. Recruitment; Retention.

Rationale. Numerous factors influence where a physician chooses to practice. Some of the factors are characteristics of the practice site or the community, such as schools or employment opportunities for a spouse (American Academy of Family Practice, 2006; Rosenblatt, et al., 2006; Casey, et al., 2005; DHSS/ACRH, 2006). Other critical factors include the population and economic base of the community that can support a physician's practice (Wright, et al., 2001). Communities that do not address such factors in their site and in their recruitment and retention efforts are less effective in securing and retaining physicians for their community. Providing tools and technical assistance to communities that tap into their unique strengths, identify weaknesses and help them strategize ways to make their community more attractive to physicians will contribute to successful outcomes.

Further Discussion. The physician shortage affects not only the quality of life of a community's citizens, but also a community's economic health. Often, the health care sector is one of the largest employers in the community. The adequacy of the health care system influences communities' ability to attract and retain business. Physician supply is correlated with economic development, expressed as real per capita gross domestic product (GDP) (Cooper, et al., 2003).

Community leaders may be unfamiliar with the nature of the physician shortage, how it could affect them locally, and the mechanisms that can increase the ability to attract and retain providers. Such mechanisms include local internships and residency training, teaching opportunities for the physicians, loan repayment and scholarships, marketing strategies, and community friendliness toward the physician and their family. Community leaders need to address elements that impede physician searches, such as the perception (whether accurate or not) that rural schools, housing or spousal employment opportunities are inadequate (American Academy of Family Practice Physicians, 2006). Major perceived barriers to recruitment include low salaries and, in rural community health centers (CHCs), cultural isolation, poor-quality schools and housing, and lack of spousal job opportunities (Rosenblatt, et al., 2006). Successful recruitment is often attributed to effectively communicating the high quality of life available in a rural community and addressing the needs of the physician's family (DHSS/ACRH, 2006).

Communities need to play an active role in assuring that there are an adequate number of providers in their communities. Since small communities often lack recruitment staff, they may benefit from training on effective recruitment strategies. Also a clear, concise description of the shortage facing Alaska can stimulate local problem solving.

Community characteristics, economic expansion and physician supply are interrelated. Major factors cited by graduating family practice residents as important ones in choosing their first medical practice site, include: significant other's wishes; medical community friendly to family physicians; recreation/culture; proximity to family/friends; significant other's employment; schools for children; size of community; initial income guarantee; benefits plan; proximity to spouse's family/friends (American Academy of Family Physicians, 2006).

Marketing strategies that highlight community resources as a component of the physician recruitment efforts need to be developed. Such marketing strategies should address factors cited by physicians such as their perceptions of community inadequacies related to schools, housing or spousal employment. Marketing the Alaska lifestyle to outside doctors is another effective strategy. (Commonwealth, 2005. p. 30).

> *"Just as we have marketed Alaskan king crab and Copper River salmon, we can market the variety of exciting opportunities available for physicians in this area."*
> —JOHN BRINGHURST, CEO, PETERSBURG MEDICAL CENTER.

It is important for community leaders to be aware of the challenges to recruitment and to tailor strategies to address these concerns. Community leaders can influence provider housing; hiring packages (leave, work schedules and continuing education); teaching responsibilities; and service opportunities (i.e. serving on local, regional, State, national committees).

Community and health care leaders must acknowledge that their communities may not have the economic capacity to support physicians or maintain state-of-the-art equipment and facilities. This situation can be caused by low population of the community, high poverty status of the community, or because the community is too geographically isolated or disadvantaged to financially support physicians. Continuous subsidies would be required to sustain a physician in such areas (Wright, et al., 2001).

A report on Kentucky's physician shortage identified a number of barriers to physician recruitment and retention. Such barriers included: medical education costs, workload and demands; and decreased opportunity for professional contacts in medically underserved areas. Economic concerns that affected recruitment and retention included: publicly supported insurance programs (Medicaid and Medicare) that reimburse rural providers at a lower rate than urban providers for the same medical procedures; rise in insurance payments; relief coverage and assurance of a reasonable amount of time off from work is the most important factor in decisions to stay or leave. Other issues include quality of public schools and ability to become a part of the local community, which was scored as more important than income. Having an unhealthy population with high rates of disease including heart disease, hypertension, asthma, diabetes and cancer can affect the ability to recruit and retain physicians (Casey, et al., 2005).

Physicians involved in teaching remain in rural practice longer than those who are not involved. Although many urban physicians assume otherwise, rural physicians do not necessarily view professional isolation and an inability to access medical information as drawbacks to rural practice. Lack of quality of rural school systems, perceived or real, is related to length of stay for physicians in a rural practice. (American Academy of Family Physicians, 2006.)

The Medical Provider Workforce Assessment Office would coordinate this strategy's activities and support existing organizations that work on physician supply and recruitment, e.g., State Office of Rural Health and Primary Care Office in DHSS; Primary Care Association, Alaska AHEC, ACRH, ANTHC, University of Alaska, ASHNA and professional associations such as ASMA. Linkages among health care sites that recruit and employ physicians, mayors, city/borough managers, tribal health corporation leadership, economic development organizations, Chambers of Commerce, the AFMR, and other training institutions need to be strengthened. Contracts with statewide organizations that address health care issues would be needed to support training events and technical assistance.

The NHSC Site Development Manual recommends the formation of a Community Primary Health Care Council that would be involved in making decisions related to the community's health care system, including developing sites that can tap into NHSC resources and providers who are NHSC Scholars or are eligible for NHSC Loan Repayment (U.S. DHHS, 2006).

Strategy 4C. Support Federal tax credit legislation initiative for physicians that meet frontier practice requirements.

Problem. There are insufficient financial incentives to attract and retain physicians in rural/frontier practices. Financial-related recruitment strategies often create non-cash income that is subject to Federal income tax.

Action Step. Engage statewide health care partners in efforts to pass physician tax credit legislation at the Federal level.

Timeframe. Short term. 12 months.

Benefit. A tax credit will help offset the taxes on the non-cash taxable income created by a loan forgiveness program and thus maintain the recruitment benefit of such programs. Additionally, when a tax liability is not a factor, a tax credit, in effect, increases the income of a physician practicing in a frontier area which influences practice location decisions.

Cost. Zero cost to the State.

Responsibility. The Alaska Congressional Delegation with support of the Alaska State Hospital and Nursing Association, ASMA, and health care partners.

Impact. Recruitment; Retention.

Rationale. Financial-related recruitment strategies that are commonly used, such as loan repayment programs, create non-cash income that is often subject to Federal income tax. A tax credit approach made available to physicians who practice in frontier areas or who treat patients from frontier areas would help maintain the recruiting benefit of a loan forgiveness program.

Further Discussion. A tax credit will help offset the taxes on the non-cash taxable income created by a loan forgiveness program and thus maintain the recruitment benefit of such programs. Additionally, when a tax liability is not a factor, a tax credit, in effect, increases the income of a physician practicing in a frontier area.

The loan forgiveness program that is currently in place for WWAMI students forgives the loan at a rate of 20 percent per year of Alaskan practice. For example, a WWAMI graduate, with $150,000 in loan repayment obligation who practices in Alaska for 5 years, has $30,000 per year in taxable income created.

S.2789 introduced on May 11, 2006 by Senator Conrad Burns (Montana) and Senator Lisa Murkowski is an example of legislation that provides for tax credits for physicians who practice in frontier areas or treat patients from frontier areas. The tax credit is $1,000 a month for a maximum 60 months. (This bill amends the Internal Revenue Code of 1986).

A short-term timeframe for adoption of such legislation is important. The WWAMI loan forgiveness element (for practice in Alaska) is impacting the first WWAMI students completing their GME this year.

This is a strategy that would not have impact on the Alaska State budget. The cost will depend on the extent of financial incentive strategies that create non-cash taxable income and the extent to which they are used. The cost is in "soft dollars" of Federal income tax not collected.

SECTION VII. AREAS THAT WARRANT FURTHER CONSIDERATION

Some areas related to Alaska's physician supply warrant further consideration but could not be discussed in depth in this report, due to limits of the Task Force's directive and time constraints. Such areas include:

- patterns and effect of physician turnover on the physician supply;
- the need for specialists and sub-specialists;
- the impact of physician assistants and advanced nurse practitioners on the need for physicians;
- the impact of community health aides on medical care in Alaska;
- the opportunities offered by the developing Doctor of Osteopathy program in Yakima, Washington;
- the factors within the Alaska practice environment that influence decisions to practice in the State;
- the relationship of the needs of subpopulations such as the elderly and those in urban as well as rural locations, on physician supply;
- the role of emerging technologies including electronic health records and tele-health in physician supply and practice; and
- the relationship between physician supply and health care access.

The Task Force determined that while many of these topics would be appropriate duties of the proposed Medical Provider Workforce Assessment Office, some of the areas would fall under the responsibilities of other organizations.

SECTION VIII. APPENDICES

A. Data Details
    1. Matriculants in Medical Schools by State
    2. Specialty Distribution Comparison (2004) Alaska and United States
B. Strategies Preferences Scoresheet
C. Physician Study Annotated Reference List
D. Resource List
E. Individual Contributors, Persons Consulted, Commentors, Reviewers, and Persons who attended Task Force Meetings
F. Acronym List

APPENDIX A. DATA DETAILS

1. Matriculants in Medical Schools by State

Applicants		Applicants' Matriculation Status					
		Matriculated In State		Matriculated Out of State		NOT Matriculated	
		N	Percent	N	Percent	N	Percent
Region							
Northeast	7,867	2,072	26.3	1,773	22.5	4,022	51.1
Central	8,580	2,884	33.6	1,125	13.1	4,571	53.3
South	12,089	4,287	35.5	1,284	10.6	6,518	53.9
West	8,069	1,439	17.8	2,041	25.3	4,589	56.9
U.S. Total	37,364	10,682	28.6	6,322	16.9	20,360	54.5
State of Legal Residence, Western States:							
Alaska	**73**			**29**	**39.7**	**44**	**60.3**
Arizona	602	109	18.1	98	16.3	395	65.6
California	4,288	812	18.9	1,167	27.2	2,309	53.8
Colorado	609	108	17.7	125	20.5	376	61.7
Hawaii	208	51	24.5	39	18.8	118	56.7
Idaho	161			61	37.9	100	62.1
Montana	108			53	49.1	55	50.9
Nevada	167	42	25.1	25	15	100	59.9
New Mexico	245	71	29	24	9.8	150	61.2
Oregon	387	68	17.6	87	22.5	232	59.9
Utah	478	75	15.7	150	31.4	253	52.9
Washington	670	103	15.4	155	23.1	412	61.5
Wyoming	73			28	38.4	45	61.6

Alaska Applicants to Medical School by Year, 1994–2005

1994	1995	1996	1997	1998	1999	2000	2001	2002	2003	2004	2005
72	51	62	59	60	48	59	76	75	69	71	73

Source: AAMC: Data Warehouse: Applicant Matriculant File as of 10/20/2005.

2. Specialty Distribution Comparison (2004), Alaska and U.S.

2004 Alaska Population: 657,755 Specialty	Alaska Total Physicians	Alaska Total Patient Care Physicians	Alaska Patient Care Phys/1,000	U.S. Patient Care Phys/1,000	Alaska "Expected # at U.S. rate"	Alaska "Actual" minus "Expected at U.S. Rate"*
Total Physicians	1,580	1347	2.05	2.38	1,569	−222
	2.28/1,000					
Primary Care	732	709	1.08	1.14	753	−44
Family Medicine	342	333	0.51	0.26	173	160
GP/FM	34	33	0.05	0.04	25	8
Internal Medicine	161	157	0.24	0.48	315	−158
Pediatrics	116	108	0.16	0.23	148	−40
Ob/Gyn	79	78	0.12	0.14	91	−13
Med Spec	57	55	0.08	0.19	126	−71
SurgSpec	243	237	0.36	0.39	259	−22
General Surgery	73	71	0.11	0.12	81	−10
Child & Adol Psych	4	3	0.00	0.02	14	−11
Psychiatry	74	66	0.10	0.13	83	−17
Emergency Medicine	75	72	0.11	0.09	60	12
OthSpec	231	205	0.31	0.40	263	−58
Neurology	12	12	0.02	0.04	28	−16
Anesthesiology	75	74	0.11	0.13	84	−10
Non Pt Care Activities	69					
Inactive	117					
Not classified	47					

Adapted by HPSD/AKDHSS
*Negative implies potential "need"

Source: AMA 2006 (Master File database)

APPENDIX B. STRATEGIES PREFERENCES SCORESHEET: STRATEGIES FOR INCREASING PHYSICIAN SUPPLY IN ALASKA

COMPLETED BY MEMBERS OF THE PHYSICIAN SUPPLY TASK FORCE (6 RESPONDENTS)

Strategy-Short Title	Strategy Description		Preference Scale (circle number reflecting your preferences, keeping in mind cost, feasibility, desirability, effectiveness)					
	Short Term (1-5 year impact on supply)	Resp 1	Resp 2	Resp 3	Resp 4	Resp 5	Resp 6	Average Response
Recruitment	Overall Recruitment Effort	3		4	4			3.7
	Targeting ad campaigns (prof. journals, TV).	3	3	3	3	2	3	2.8
	Recruitment at national meetings of the specialty societies.	3	5	3	3	5	4	3.8
	Match candidates with local cultural and recreational needs.	3	3	3	2	4	3	3.0
	Include spouse/SO and family in recruitment.	4	5	3	5	5	3	4.2
	Use recruiters from the local area	3	4	2	4	5	3	3.5
	Explain advantages of work in underserved areas, rural communities.	2	4	3	3	3	3	3.0
	Signing bonuses	2	5	4	4	5	5	4.2
	Loan repayment options available	4	3	4	5	5	5	4.3
	Higher salary and benefit offerings (including leave options).	4		4	5	5	3	4.2
	Tax credits	2		5	5	5	5	4.4
Retention	Overall Retention Effort	4		4	4			4.0
	Provide extra support to integrate provider and family into local community.	3	4	4	4	3	3	3.5
	Loan repayment options available	4	5	4	5	5	5	4.7
	Improved salary and benefit scales.	4	4	4	4	5	4	4.2
	Offer/improve housing		3	4	5	2	3	3.4
	Improved clinical facilities		4	3	3	3	2	3.0
	Good schools/community resources	5	4	4	5	4	4	4.3
Practice environment.	Overall Practice Environment Effort.	1		3	4			2.7
	Continuing education opportunities			2	4	2	3	2.8
	Good management in work environment.			3	4	2	3	3.0
	More opportunity for professional interaction thru videoconferencing & other means.			1	4	3	3	2.8
	Welcome provider to community ...			2	4		2	2.7
	Flexible schedule and call			2	3	3	3	2.8
	Malpractice insurance relief/support.			3	4	4	1	3.0
	Adequate staffing			3	5	2	2	3.0
Education/ Training.	Overall Education/Training Effort ..	5		5	4			4.7
	Expand residency programs	5	5	5	5	4	5	4.8
	Increase medical school slots	5	5	5	5	5	5	5.0
	Early college conditioning for health careers.	4	5	4	4	3	5	4.2
	Pre-college	3	5	3	4	3	3	3.5

Strategy-Short Title	Strategy Description		Preference Scale (circle number reflecting your preferences, keeping in mind cost, feasibility, desirability, effectiveness)						
	Short Term (1-5 year impact on supply)	Resp 1	Resp 2	Resp 3	Resp 4	Resp 5	Resp 6	Average Response
	AHEC program expansion	3	5	2	3	3	5	3.5
	Mentor Alaskan high school students to be health providers—talk at local schools.	3	5	2	3	3	3	3.2
	Scholarships	4	5	3	5	4	4	4.2

Medium Term (6–20 year planning horizon)

Strategy-Short Title	Strategy Description	Resp 1	Resp 2	Resp 3	Resp 4	Resp 5	Resp 6	Average Response
Education/ Training								
	Medical school in Alaska	5	2	4	2	4	2	3.2
	Additional medical school slots	5	5	5	4	5	5	4.8
Practice environment.	Additional residency programs	5	5	4	5	4	5	4.7
Retention	New and improved healthcare facilities.	4	4	3	4	3	3	3.5
Financial Incentives.	Improved housing and facilities ...	3	4	3	4	2	2	3.0
	Improved health insurance coverage.	2	4	3	3	1	2	2.5

Long Term (>20 years)

Strategy-Short Title	Strategy Description	Resp 1	Resp 2	Resp 3	Resp 4	Resp 5	Resp 6	Average Response
Education/ Training.								
	Medical school in Alaska	5	5	5	2	4	5	4.3

APPENDIX C. PHYSICIAN STUDY ANNOTATED REFERENCE LIST

Casey, B.R, Jones, J., Gross, D.A., Dixon, L. (2004). Rural Kentucky's physician shortage: strategies for producing, recruiting and retaining primary care providers within a medically underserved region. Revised for publication in the *Journal of the Kentucky Medical Association*, September 2005. University of Kentucky, Center for Rural Health.
http://www.mc.uky.edu/RuralHealth/Research/WhitePaperJKMArvsd.pdf.

Kentucky has 400 family physicians that are age 60 or above. The State's rural medical residency programs can produce only 16 to 18 new family physicians each year. The number of residency applications has decreased in recent years. Strategies: addition of an osteopathic medical school, rural residency programs, State support for family practice GME, physician placement services, State loan repayment program, J-1 Visa, reform medical liability.

Center for Health Workforce Studies, University at Albany, State University of New York. (2004). *California physician workforce: supply and demand through 2015.*
http://www.ucop.edu/healthaffairs/reports/Final%20Report%20-%20California%20Physician%20Workforce_12_20042.pdf.

California is likely to face a 5 percent–16 percent shortage of physicians by 2015. Some communities are likely to experience more serious shortages than others. Strategies to address projected shortages and mal-distribution include: (1) increasing the supply by increasing medical school capacity, graduate medical training capacity, incentives to encourage migration to the State and to retain physicians currently practicing in the State; (2) increasing the productivity and capacity of the existing physician workforce by expanding the supply and use of non-physician clinicians, new technologies and increasing the use of treatment protocols and utilization review; (3) increasing the diversity of the physician workforce; (4) promoting a more effective environment for physician workforce planning and policies by increasing data collection and monitoring physician requirements, tracking physician supply, comprehensive re-assessment every 5 years, statewide process for physician workforce planning; (5) promoting programs and policies such as identification and publication of shortage areas by specialty, physician loan-repayment and placement, targeted site development grants, medical education and training in shortage areas, increasing reimbursement rates in shortage areas.

Chen, F.M., Fordyce, M.A, Hart, L.G. (2005). *WWAMI physician workforce 2005.* WWAMI Center for Health Workforce Studies, Working Paper #98.
http://www.fammed.washington.edu/CHWS/reports/CHWSWP98%20Chen.pdf.

The UWSOM currently produces approximately 175 physicians a year and over 60 percent of graduating students stay within the five-state area to practice. Almost 50 percent of graduating students pursue careers in primary care. Twenty percent of WWAMI graduates will practice in federally-designated Health Professional Shortage Areas. This analysis utilized the 2005 AMA Master File to determine the population-based supply of physicians at the State and county level, by discipline of physician and whether they graduated or trained at UWSOM. Currently there are 22,578 physicians in the five-state WWAMI region. Of these, 18,794 are clinically-active. Two-thirds (12,718) are in Washington. Wyoming has the smallest number (830).

Council on Graduate Medical Education. (2005). *Seventeenth report: minorities in medicine: an ethnic and cultural challenge for physician training.*
http://www.cogme.gov/17thReport/17.htm.

Findings: "Family income" is the most influential factor in determining whether a high school senior will be "very well qualified" for college, based on class rank, grade point average and scores on standardized tests. Parents' education and income levels affect academic achievement of children. Disproportionate numbers of "underrepresented minority" children live in single-parent and low-income households. Although some programs promote children's interest, academic achievement, and career choices in science and health, a need exists for organizations to partner with media, advertising and marketing firms to develop and disseminate culturally appropriate messages targeted to minority and disadvantaged youth to encourage academic persistence and achievement and interest in medical careers.

Council on Graduate Medical Education. (2005). *Sixteenth report: physician workforce policy guidelines for the United States, 2000–2020.*
http://www.cogme.gov/pubs.htm.

The supply of practicing physicians is expected to rise 24 percent from 781,200 to 971,800 between 2000 and 2020. Growth is expected to slow after 2010 due to the aging of the workforce and the relatively level number of new physician entrants since 1980. At the same time the demand for physicians is likely to grow more rapidly than the supply and the need for services is expected to increase. Considering supply and need, a shortage of 96,000 is projected in 2020. Factors, such as changing lifestyles, increase in the use and expected increases in the Nation's wealth, are included in this report. Other factors not included are: potential increase in non-patient care activities, change in practice patterns for physicians over 50, departures due to liability concerns, limiting the number of patients ("boutique medicine") and individuals with chronic illnesses living longer.

Council on Graduate Medical Education. (1998) *Tenth report: physician distribution and health care challenges in rural and inner-city areas.*
http://www.cogme.gov/rpt10.htm.

Findings include the following: The lack of health insurance presents the greatest barrier to medical care. Safety net programs such as CHCs and the NHSC are essential mechanisms for insuring access to health care for underserved populations. Growth in the number of physicians in the United States has not eliminated the problem of geographic mal-distribution. The small number of family physicians has contributed to the shortage of rural physicians. PAs and ANPs play an important role in providing medical care in rural underserved areas. CHCs and group practice arrangements may be the most viable model for increasing care in underserved areas.

Grumbach K., Coffman, J.M., Young, J.Q., Vranizan, K., Blick, N. (1998). *Physician supply and medical education in California: a comparison with national trends.* University of California, San Francisco, Medical School, Department of Family and Community Medicine.
http://www.pubmedcentral.nih.gov/articlerender.fcgi?artid=1304984.

This study concluded that California has an ample supply of physicians in the aggregate, but too many specialists, too few underrepresented racial/ethnic minority physicians, and poor distribution of physicians across the State. These factors will continue to exert inflationary pressures on the health care system without improving access to care. Major policy changes are needed to address the imbalance.

Grumbach, K., Coffman, J., Liu, R., Mertz, E. (1999). Strategies for increasing physician supply in medically underserved communities in California. California Policy Research Center Brief Series, Center for California Health Workforce Studies.
http://www.ucop.edu/cprc/MDsupply.html.

This report recommends three types of strategies to increase the physician supply in underserved areas: (1) practice-environment to make practice in shortage areas more attractive (2) medical education to address the training experiences of physicians (3) applicant pool to target the types of students who enter medical school. Practice-environment interventions have the quickest "pay off" in improving physician distribution because they target the point when physicians are ready to enter practice. Medical education and applicant-pool strategies are integral to a comprehensive plan but take longer to yield results.

Hart, L.G., Lishner, D.M., Larson, E.H., Chen, C., Andrilla, H.A., Norris, T.E., Schneeweiss, R., Henderson, T.M. and Rosenblatt, R.A. (2005). Pathways to rural practice: a chart book of family medicine residency training locations and characteristics. *http://www.ask.hrsa.gov/detail.cfm?PublD=ORHP00324.*

A survey of U.S. family medicine residencies was conducted in January 2000. Of the 453 questionnaires sent, 435 responded (96 percent). Only 33 of the responding programs (7.6 percent) were located in rural areas; predominantly in community hospitals. Over one-third of the urban programs listed rural training as an important part of their mission; however, only 2.3 percent of their training took place in rural areas. For the Nation as a whole, 7.5 percent of family medicine residency training occurred within rural areas, although 22.3 percent of the U.S. population lives in rural places. The number of rural residencies has declined since the survey was conducted. Unless significant efforts are made to increase rural residency training, rural physician shortages are likely to persist.

Institute of Medicine of the National Academies. (2005). *Quality through collaboration: the future of rural health care.* National Academies Press.

This report discussed improvements in the three broad areas of the pipeline to increase the size of a quality rural workforce: (1) attracting rural students to health careers, (2) providing formal education programs, and (3) recruiting and retaining trained health professionals in rural areas. (p. 89)

Measures to attract rural students to health careers involve enrichment of schooling for pre-collegiate students, ensuring that basic science is part of the curriculum, and ensuring that students have positive exposure to role models and career paths in rural health care delivery. (p. 91)

It is important to create opportunities for members of minority and disadvantaged populations. Programs administered by HRSA and improved admissions processes can assist in this effort. (p. 93)

For physicians, two factors are strongly predictive of a future career in rural health: a rural background and plans to enter family medicine. (Rabinowitz and Taylor, 2004). Medical schools that make a strong commitment to educating physicians for rural practice quite successful track records. (p. 94)

Ricketts, T.C. (2005). Workforce issues in rural areas: a focus on policy equity. *American Journal of Public Health*, 95, 42–48.
http://www.ajph.org/cgi/content/abstract/95/1/42.

Rural communities in the United States are served by fewer health care professionals than urban or suburban areas. This review of the geographic distribution of health professionals and policies and programs that influence practice location decisions identifies three categories of policy levers: coercive, normative and utilitarian; and recommends a balanced use of the three approaches.

Southworth, M. (2004). *Alaskan's physician workforce: an overview, a summary of training backgrounds, and the impact of the WWAMI program.* Thesis submitted for degree of Master of Public Health, University of Washington.

Alaska has 1,304 physicians with an active Alaska medical license that were reviewed. 93.7 percent MD degrees, 6.3 percent DO degrees; 76.6 percent at least one board certification; 30.2 percent women; 24.6 percent addresses in rural communities; osteopaths 1.6 percent of rural physicians and 4.6 percent of urban physicians; women 34.3 percent rural and 28.8 percent urban; generalists 43.7 percent; surgical 21.9 percent; medical specialists 8.0 percent; other fields 26.4 percent; 29 percent fewer generalists per 100,000 population in rural communities. 9.9 percent of Alaska physicians received degrees at UWSOM; 9.6 percent from four other schools; 9.4 percent U.S. military postgraduate training. 52.6 percent of UWSOM graduates are generalists and 24.1 percent are in rural communities. Alaska's physician workforce is growing but geographically mal-distributed.

Taylor, P. *Utah links Federal funding for graduate medical education to State's physician workforce needs.* Publication produced for U.S. Department of Health and Human Services, Health Resources & Services Administration, Office of Rural Health Policy. *http://ruralhealth.hrsa.gov/pub/UtahGME.asp.*

A state-chartered commission in Utah is linking Utah's GME funding and statewide physician workforce needs. The Medicare GME demonstration project gives the Utah Medical Education Council authority to receive and disburse all Utah Medicare Direct Medical Education payments. One goal of the demonstration is to increase the number of graduating physicians who choose to practice in rural areas.

U.S. Department of Health and Human Services, Health Resources and Services Administration, Bureau of Health Professions, National Center for Health Workforce Analysis. (Spring 2003). *Changing demographics: implications for physicians, nurses, and other health workers.*
http://bhpr.hrsa.gov/healthworkforce/reports/changedemo/default.htm.

The findings of the literature and two demand forecasting models: the Physician Aggregate Requirements Model (PARM) and the Nursing Demand Model (NDM) are: aging population will increase the demand for physicians per 1,000 from 2.8 in 2000 to 3.1 in 2020. Between 2000 and 2020 the percentage of patient care hours spent with minority patients will rise from 31 to 40 percent. Increases under five scenarios are projected: status quo (33 percent), baseline (28 percent), universal coverage (40 percent), 100 percent HMO (36 percent) and non-minority rates (37 percent).

U.S. General Accounting Office (October 2003). *Physician workforce: physician supply increased in metropolitan and non-metropolitan areas but geographic disparities persisted.* Report to the Chairman, Committee on Health, Education, Labor, and Pensions, U.S. Senate. GAO-04-124. *http://www.gao.gov/new.items/d04124.pdf.*

The GAO analyzed data on physician supply and geographic distribution from 1991 and 2001. The U.S. physician population increased 26 percent, which was twice the rate of total population growth, between 1991 and 2001. The average number of physicians per 100,000 people increased from 214 to 239 and the mix of generalists and specialists in the national physician workforce remained about one-third generalists and two-thirds specialists. Non-metropolitan counties with a large town (10,000 to 49,000 residents) had the biggest increase in physicians per 100,000 people of all county categories but their supplies were still less than large and small metropolitan counties in 1991 and 2001.

Utah Medical Education Council, State of Utah. (2006). *Utah 's physician workforce: a study on the supply and distribution of physicians in Utah.*
http://www.utahmec.org/physicians.htm.

The UMEC conducted a survey of all State licensed physicians. Of 4,484 physicians working in Utah only 3,894 were active patient care providers. The characteristics of the Utah physician workforce mirror the national workforce. Over 55 percent of the physicians practicing in Utah had had some previous contact with the State. Only 12 percent of Utah physicians provide services to the 25 rural counties in the State. Utah will need to recruit up to 270 physicians per year to meet the projected demand.

Wisconsin Hospital Association and the Wisconsin Medical Society. (2004). Who will care for our patients? Wisconsin takes action to fight a growing physician shortage.
http://www.wha.org/physicianshortage3-04.pdf.

There is a shortage of primary care physicians in rural Wisconsin and inner city Milwaukee. Non-primary specialty physicians are in demand and are hard to recruit on a statewide basis. General surgeons and radiologists are critically needed in rural areas. The unmet needs are projected to grow. By 2015, demand is expected to increase by 13.5 percent for primary care physicians and 20 percent for all other physicians. Action plan: enroll students, develop new care delivery models, attract and retain physicians, enhance funding, create a medical education infrastructure.

APPENDIX D. RESOURCE LIST

Alaska Department of Health and Social Services, Office of the Commissioner, Health Planning and Systems Development, and University of Alaska Anchorage Center for Rural Health. (2006). *Status of recruitment resources and strategies.* *http://hss.state.ak.us/commissioner/healthplanning/publications.*

Alexander, C., Fraser, J., Simpkins, B., Temperley, J. (2003). Health career promotion in the New England area of New South Wales: a program to support high school career advisers. *Australian Journal of Rural Health*, 11(4):199–204.

American Academy of Family Physicians. *Rural practice, keeping physicians in. (Position Paper).* (Retrieved 6/7/2006). *http://www.aafp.org/online/en/home/policy/policies/r/ruralpracticekeep.html.*

American Medical Association, Center for Health Policy Research. (2003). *Physician socioeconomic statistics 2001*, Tables 13 and 14.

Association of American Medical Colleges, Center for Workforce Studies. (2006). *Key Physician Data by State. http://www.aamc.org/workforce/statedata.pdf.*

Association of American Medical Colleges. (2004). *COGME report predicts physician shortage. http://www.aamc.org/newsroom/reporter/nov04/cogme.htm.*

Association of American Medical Colleges. (2004). *Rural medicine programs aim to reverse physician shortage in outlying regions.* *http://www.aamc.org/newsroom/reporter/nov04/rural.htm.*

Association of American Medical Colleges. (2006). Notes from conference May 4–5, 2006. *Physician Workforce Research Conference: 2020 Vision—Focusing on the Future.*

Bacon T.J., Baden D.J., Coccodrilli L.D. (2000). The national area health education center program and primary care residency training. *Journal of Rural Health*, 16(3):288–294.

Barrans, D. (2006). *Alaskan participation in the WICHE professional student exchange program.* Memorandum to members of Alaska Physician Supply Task Force. Alaska Advantage Programs, Alaska Commission on Postsecondary Education.

Booker, J.M., Garrett, C. and Helmuth, B. (1995). *A survey of primary care providers in Alaska.*

Boulger J.G. (2000). Stability of practice location among UMD family physicians in Minnesota. *Minnesota Medicine.* 83(2):48–50.

Bowman, R.C. (2005). *Bright future rankings.* University of Nebraska Medical Center. *www.unmc.edu/Community/ruralmeded/bright_future_rankings.htm.*

Bowman, R.C. (2005). *Flawed physician workforce "beliefs." University of Nebraska Medical Center.* *www.unmc.edu/Community/ruralmeded/flawed_physician_workforce.htm.*

Bowman, R.C. (2005). *Medical school expansion 2004–2017.* University of Nebraska Medical Center. *www.unmc.edu/Community/ruralmeded/expansion_medical_schools.htm.*

Bowman, R.C. *Physician distribution in the United States.* University of Nebraska Medical Center. (Retrieved 4/5/2006) *www.unmc.edu/Community/ruralmeded/physician_distribution_in_the_us.htm.*

Bowman, R.C. (2005). *Ranking medical schools and FP residency programs.* University of Nebraska Medical Center. *http://www.unmc.edu/Community/ruralmeded/ranking_rural.htm.*

Casey, B.R, Jones, J., Gross, D.A., Dixon, L. (2004). Rural Kentucky's physician shortage: strategies for producing, recruiting and retaining primary care providers within a medically underserved region. Revised for publication in the *Journal of the Kentucky Medical Association*, September 2005. University of Kentucky, Center for Rural Health. *http://www.mc.uky.edu/RuralHealth/Research/WhitePaperJKMArvsd.pdf.*

Cejka Search. (2005). *Physician shortage assessments should reflect economics rather than demographics. http://www.cejkasearch.com/news/default.htm.*

Center for Health Policy, Research & Ethics. (2000). *The National Health Service Corps: "essential" but unseen.* George Mason University, Fairfax, Virginia.

Center for Health Workforce Studies, University at Albany, State University of New York. (2004). *California physician workforce: supply and demand through 2015.* *http://www.ucop.edu/healthaffairs/reports/Final%20Report%20-%20California%20Physician%20Workforce_12_20042.pdf.*

Chan, B.T.B., Degani, N., Chrichton, T., Pong, R.W., Rourke, J.T., Goertzen, J., McCready, B. (2005). Factors influencing family physicians to enter rural practice. *Canadian Family Physician*, vol. 51. *http://www.cfpc.ca/cfp/2005/Sep/vol51-sep-research-5.asp.*

Chen, F.M., Fordyce, M.A, Hart, L.G. (2005). *WWAMI physician workforce 2005.* WWAMI Center for Health Workforce Studies, Working Paper #98. *http://www.fammed.washington.edu/CHWS/reports/CHWSWP98%20Chen.pdf.*

CHAP Directors' Association. (2001). *Community health aide program update 2001: Alaska's rural health care at risk.* Final report for the Alaska Native Health Board and the Association of Tribal Health Directors.

Cooper, R.A. (2004). Medicine and public issues: weighing the evidence for expanding physician supply. *Annals of Internal Medicine*, 141(9), 705–711. *http://www.annals.org.*

Cooper, R.A. (2002). There's a shortage of specialists. Is anyone listening? *Academic Medicine*, 77 (8), 761–766.

Cooper, R.A., Getzen, T.E., Laud, P. (2003). Economic expansion is a major determinant of physician supply and utilization. *Health Services Research*, 38(2).

Cooper, R.A., Getzen, T.E., McKee, H.J., Laud, P. (2002). Economic and demographic trends signal an impending physician shortage. *Health Affairs*, 21(1), 140–154.

Council on Graduate Medical Education. (1998). *Tenth report: physician distribution and health care challenges in rural and inner-city areas.* *http://www.cogme.gov/rpt10.htm.*

Council on Graduate Medical Education. (2005). *Sixteenth report: physician workforce policy guidelines for the United States, 2000–2020.* *http//www.cogme.gov/pubs.htm.*

Council on Graduate Medical Education. (2005). *Seventeenth report: minorities in medicine: an ethnic and cultural challenge for physician training.* *http://www.cogme.gov/17thReport/17.htm.*

Elder N, Taylor A, Anderson CE, Virgin R. (1997). Health career orientation of Oregon high school students. *Family Medicine*, 29(2):108–11.

Foster, M, Goldsmith, S. (2006). Alaska's $5 billion health care bill—who's paying? *Understanding Alaska: UA Research Summary No. 6*, Institute of Social and Economic Research, University of Alaska, Anchorage. *http://www.alaskaneconomy.uaa.alaska.edu.*

Green, L.A., Phillips, R.L. (2005). The family physician workforce: quality, not quantity. *American Family Physician*, 71 (12), 2248–2253. *http://www.aafp/org/afp.*

Grumbach K., Coffman, J.M., Young, J.Q., Vranizan, K., Blick, N. (1998). *Physician supply and medical education in California: a comparison with national trends.* University of California, San Francisco, Medical School, Department of Family and Community Medicine. *http://www.pubmedcentral.nih.gov/articlerender.fcgi?artid=1304984.*

Grumbach, K., Coffman, J., Liu, R., Mertz, E. (1999). Strategies for increasing physician supply in medically underserved communities in California. *California Policy Research Center Brief Series, Center for California Health Workforce Studies.* *http://www.ucop.edu/cprc/MDsupply.html.*

Hager, C., *Update on NCHWA Models and Activities.* PowerPoint Presentation. National Center for Workforce Analysis, Bureau of Health Professions, HRSA. (6/1/2006).

Hagopian, A., Thompson, M.J., Kaltenbach, E., Hart, L.G. (2003). Health departments' use of international medical graduates in physician shortage areas. *Health Affairs*, 22 (5), 241–249.

Schneeweiss, R., Henderson, T.M. and Rosenblatt, R.A. (2005). *Pathways to rural practice: a chart book of family medicine residency training locations and characteristics. http://www.ask.hrsa.gov/detail.cfm?PubID=ORHP00324.*

Henderson, T.M. (2003). *Medicaid direct and indirect graduate medical education payments: a 50-state survey.* Association of American Medical Colleges. *http://www.aamc.org.*

Heyman, D., (Ed.), Kiley, D. (Hartig Fellow). (2005). *Alaska primary health care: opportunities and challenges.* Commonwealth North. *www.commonwealthnorth.org.*

Institute of Medicine of the National Academies, Committee on the Future of Rural Health Care. (2005). *Quality through collaboration: the future of rural health care.*

Foster, M. and Goldsmith, S. (2006). Alaskan's $5 billion health care bill—who's paying? *Understanding Alaska*. Institute of Social and Economic Research, University of Alaska Anchorage. UA Research Summary No, 6. *www.uaa.alaskaneconomy.uaa.alaska.edu*.

Jones A, Oster R, Pederson L, Kidd-Davis M, Blumenthal D. (2000). Influence of a Rural Primary Care Clerkship on Medical Students' Intentions to Practice in a Rural Community. *The Journal of Rural Health*, 16(2): 155–161.

Lewin Group. (2006). *Data and methods for forecasting physician demand*. 2006 AAMC Pre-conference Session presented by Tim Dall, May 3, 2006.

Massachusetts Medical Society. (2005). *Physician workforce study*. *http://www.massmed.org*.

National Rural Health Association. (1998). Physician recruitment and retention. Issue paper for NRHA. *http://www.nrharural.org/advocacy/sub/issuepapers/ipaper13.html*.

National Rural Health Association. (2005). Recruitment and Retention of a Quality Health Workforce in Rural Areas. *NRHA Issue Paper*. *http://www.nrharural.org/advocacy/sub/issuepapers/ipaperl3.html*

National Rural Recruitment and Retention Network (3RNet). (2006). *http://www.3RNet.org*.

Neill J, Taylor K. (2002). Undergraduate nursing students' clinical experiences in rural and remote areas: recruitment implications. *Australian Journal of Rural Health*, 10(5):239–243.

Pathman, D.E., Konrad, T.R., King. T.S., Taylor, D.H., Koch, G.G. (2004). Outcomes of states' scholarship, loan repayment, and related programs for physicians. *Medical Care*, 42(6).

Physician Compensation Report. (2003). *COGME favors slow growth in med schools, residencies*.

Rabinowitz, H, Diamond, J, Veloski, J.J., & Gayle, J.A. (2000). The impact of multiple predictors on generalist physicians' care of underserved populations. *American Journal of Public Health*, 90(8): 1225–1228.

Rabinowitz, H.K., Diamond, J.J., Markham, F.W., Hazelwood, C.E. (1999). Physician Shortage Area Program (PSAP). Jefferson Medical. *Journal of the American Medical Association*, College 281:255–260.

Ramsey, P.G., Coombs J.B., Hunt D.D. (2001). From concept to culture: the WWAMI Program at the University of Washington School of Medicine. *Academic Medicine*, 76(8):756–778.

Ricketts, T.C. (2005). Workforce issues in rural areas: a focus on policy equity. *American Journal of Public Health*, 95, 42–48. *http://www.ajph.org/cgi/content/abstract/95/1/42*.

Rockey, P.H. (2005). *Fixing the U.S. Physician Shortage Requires many More Slots for Resident Physicians in Training*. Retrieved 5/31/06. Medscape General Medicine Webcast Video Editorial, posted May 22, 2005. *http://www.medscape.com/viewarticle/532152?src=mp*.

Rosenblatt, R.A., Andrilla, C.H.A., Curtin, T., and Hart, L.G. (2006). Shortages of medical personnel at community health centers: implications for planned expansion. *Journal of the American Medical Society*. 295(9): 1042–1049.

Salsberg, E. (2004). Council on Graduate Medical Education (COGME), AAMC Center for Workforce Studies.

Scalise, D. (2005). Physician supply 2005. *Hospitals and Health Networks*, 79(11):59–65.

Schiff, E. (2006). *Preparing the health workforce*. Issue Paper for Secretary of Education's Commission of the Future of Higher Education.

Southworth, M. (2004). *Alaskan's physician workforce: an overview, a summary of training backgrounds, and the impact of the WWAMI program*. Thesis submitted for degree of Master of Public health, University of Washington.

Taylor, P. *Utah links Federal funding for graduate medical education to State's physician workforce needs*. Publication produced for U.S. Department of Health and Human Services, Health Resources & Services Administration, Office of Rural Health Policy. *http://ruralhealth.hrsa.gov/pub/UtahGME.asp*. Retrieved March, 2006.

The U.S. News and World Report. (2006). *America's best graduate schools, 2007 edition*. *http://www.usnews.com/usnews/edu/grad/rankings/med/brief/mdprank_brief.php*.

U.S. Department of Health and Human Services, Health Resources and Services Administration, Bureau of Health Professions, National Center for Health Workforce Analysis. (2003). *Changing demographics: implications for physicians, nurses, and other health workers.* *http://bhpr.hrsa.gov/healthworkforce/reports/changedemo/default.htm.*

U.S. Department of Health and Human Services, Health Resources and Services Administration Bureau of Health Professions, National Center for Health Workforce Analysis. (2005). *Public health workforce study.* *http://bhpr.hrsa.gov/healthworkforce/reports/publichealth/default.htm.*

U.S. Department of Health and Human Services, Health Resources and Services Administration, Bureau of Health Professions, National Center for Health Workforce Analysis State Health Workforce Profiles Highlights Alaska. *The Alaska health workforce: highlights from the health workforce profile.* Retrieved 12/21/05. *http://bhpr.hrsa.gov/healthworkforce/reports/statesummaries/alaska.htm.*

U.S. Department of Health and Human Services, Health Resources and Services Administration, National Health Service Corps. (2006). *Site development manual.* *http://nhsc.bhpr.hrsa.gov/resources/SDM-toc.asp.*

U.S. General Accounting Office. (2003). *Physician workforce: physician supply increased in metropolitan and non-metropolitan areas but geographic disparities persisted.* Report to the Chairman, Committee on Health, Education, Labor, and Pensions, U.S. Senate. GAO-04-124. *http://www.gao.gov/new.items/dO4124.pdf.*

Utah Medical Education Council, State of Utah. (2006). *Utah 's physician workforce: a study on the supply and distribution of physicians in Utah.* *http://www.utahmec.org/physicians.htm.*

Western Interstate Commission for Higher Education. (2006). Opportunities for undergraduate study available to residents of participating western States *WUE Western Undergraduate Exchange 2006–2007 Bulletin.* *http://www.wiche.edu/sep/wue.*

Wisconsin Hospital Association and the Wisconsin Medical Society. (2004). *Who will care for our patients? Wisconsin takes action to fight a growing physician shortage.* *http://www.wha.org/physicianshortage3-04.pdf.*

Williams, G. (2005). Population projections: projections for Alaska population 2005–2029. *Alaska Economic Trends, February 2005.* *http://labor.state.ak.us/trends/feb05.pdf.*

Williams, G. (2005). *Alaska Department of Labor & Workforce Development releases State, borough and place 2005 population.* Media Release AKDOL No. 06-30, January 25, 2006. *http://almis.labor.state.ak.us/?PAGEID=67&SUBID=171.*

Wright, G.E., Andrilla, C.A. and Hart, G.L. (2001). *How many physicians can a rural community support?* WWAMI Rural Health Research Working Paper #45. University of Washington, School of Medicine, Department of Family Medicine. *http://depts.Washington.edu/uwrhrc/.*

WWAMI Rural Health Research Center. (2005). *Family physician vacancies in federally funded health centers.* *http://depts.washington.edu/uwrhrc/.*

APPENDIX E. INDIVIDUAL CONTRIBUTORS, PERSONS CONSULTED, COMMENTERS, REVIEWERS, AND PERSONS WHO ATTENDED TASK FORCE MEETINGS

Diane Barrans, Executive Director, Alaska Commission on Post-Secondary Education

John F. Bringhurst, CEO, Petersburg Medical Center

Liz Connell, Legislative Assistant, Office of Senator Ted Stevens

John Coombs, MD, MNS, University of Washington School of Medicine, WWAMI

Paul Davis, MD, Alaska Family Medicine Residency

Gar Elison, Executive Director, and staff, Utah Medical Education Council

Leslie Gallant, Executive Administrator, Alaska State Medical Board

Tim Gilbert, MPH, Alaska Native Tribal Health Consortium

Jan Harris, MA, MSHA, UAA, School of Nursing

Gary Hart, Ph.D., Fred Chen, MD, Eric Larson, Ph.D., UW Rural Health Research Center

Tom Hunt, MD, Medical Director, Anchorage Neighborhood Health Center

Marilyn Kasmar, RNC, MBA, Executive Director, Alaska Primary Care Association, and staff members Pat Fedrick and Richard Moore, PA-C

Beth Landon, MBA, MHA, Director, Alaska Center for Rural Health

Peter Marshall, MD, private practice, North Pole. Chairman, Alaska WWAMI Admissions Committee

Kathy Murray, BA, MLS, AHIP, UAA Health Sciences Library

Richard L. Neubauer, MD, Internal Medicine

Tom Nighswander, MD, WWAMI Program and ANMC

Theresa and Tom Obermeyer, JD, Anchorage

Byron Perkins, D.O., Association President, Alaska Osteopathic Medical Association

Tom Ricketts, Ph.D., University of North Carolina, Sheps Center

John Riley, MS, PA-C, Alaska MEDEX Program

Meredith Sumpter, Legislative Correspondent, Office of Lisa Murkowski

Leif Thompson, MD, Bristol Bay Area Health Corporation

Suzanne Tryck, Alaska WWAMI Coordinator

APPENDIX F. ACRONYM LIST

3RNET	Rural Recruitment and Retention Network
AA	Active License Status
AAHC	Alaskans for Access to Health Care (ACCESS)
AAMC	Association of American Medical Colleges
ACRH	Alaska Center for Rural Health
AFMR	Alaska Family Medicine Residency
AHEC	Area Health Education Center
AKDHSS	Alaska Department of Health and Social Services
AKOMA	Alaska Osteopathic Medical Association
AMA	American Medical Association
ANMC	Alaska Native Medical Center
ANTHC	Alaska Native Tribal Health Consortium
APCA	Alaska Primary Care Association
APCO	Alaska Primary Care Office
ASHNA	Alaska State Hospital and Nursing Home Association
ASMA	Alaska State Medical Association
AP&S	Alaska Physicians and Surgeons
BHPr	Bureau of Health Professions
CEO	Chief Executive Officer
CEU	Continuing Education Units
CHC	Community Health Center
COGME	Council of Graduate Medical Education
DHSS	Department of Health and Social Services
DO	Doctor of Osteopathy
FTE	Full Time Equivalent
GDP	Gross Domestic Product
GME	Graduate Medical Education
GMENAC	Graduate Medical Education National Advisory Committee
HMO	Health Maintenance Organization
HPSA	Health Professional Shortage Area
HPSD	Health Planning and Systems Development
HRSA	Health Resources and Services Administration
IHS	Indian Health Service
LRP	Loan Repayment Program
MD	Allopathic Physician
MMS	Massachusetts Medical Society
MNS	Master in Nutritional Science
MPH	Masters in Public Health
MUA	Medically Underserved Areas
NHSC	National Health Service Corps
OHSU	Oregon Health and Science University
PSAP	Physician Shortage Area Program
PSEP	Professional Student Exchange Program
R/UOP	Rural/Underserved Opportunities Program
SEARCH	Student/Resident Experiences and Rotations in Community Health
SLRP	State Loan Repayment Program
UA	University of Alaska
UAA	University of Alaska Anchorage
U.S. DHHS	United States Department of Health and Human Services
WICHE	Western Interstate Commission on Higher Education
WWAMI	Washington, Wyoming, Alaska, Montana, and Idaho (regional school of medicine based at the University of Washington)

(For more information on Securing an Adequate Number of Physicians for Alaska's Needs, a Report of the Alaska Physician Supply Task Force, contact: Pat Carr, Health Planning and Systems Development, (907) 465–8618, pat_carr@health.state.ak.us. This report is also available on the Web: http://www.hss.state.ak.us/commissioner/PhysicianSupply.htm.)

[Whereupon, at 12:00 p.m., the hearing was adjourned.]

○

APEX
TP_CF

765523826—47